Hamlet Hayrapetyan

Right Ventricular Infarction: Prognostic Importance of Echocardiography

AF153332

Hamlet Hayrapetyan

Right Ventricular Infarction: Prognostic Importance of Echocardiography

LAP LAMBERT Academic Publishing

Imprint

Any brand names and product names mentioned in this book are subject to trademark, brand or patent protection and are trademarks or registered trademarks of their respective holders. The use of brand names, product names, common names, trade names, product descriptions etc. even without a particular marking in this work is in no way to be construed to mean that such names may be regarded as unrestricted in respect of trademark and brand protection legislation and could thus be used by anyone.

Cover image: www.ingimage.com

Publisher:
LAP LAMBERT Academic Publishing
is a trademark of
Dodo Books Indian Ocean Ltd. and OmniScriptum S.R.L publishing group

120 High Road, East Finchley, London, N2 9ED, United Kingdom
Str. Armeneasca 28/1, office 1, Chisinau MD-2012, Republic of Moldova, Europe
Managing Directors: Ieva Konstantinova, Victoria Ursu
info@omniscriptum.com

Printed at: see last page
ISBN: 978-3-659-54481-1

In Loving Memory of My Darling Wife,
Narine Tadevosyan

Right Ventricular Myocardial Infarction: Prognostic Importance of Echocardiographic Parameters

Hamlet G. Hayrapetyan, FESC, MD

The Table of Contents

Abbreviations

ACCs – acute cardiac complications
AH – arterial hypertension
AV – atrio-ventricular
CMR – cardiac magnetic resonance
COPD – chronic obstructive pulmonary diseases
CS – cardiogenic shock
Cx – circumflex
DM – Diabetes Miletus
DMI – Doppler myocardial imaging
ECG – electrocardiography
EchoCG – echocardiography
EF – ejection fraction
ET – ejection time
FAC – fractional area change
HB – heart block
HF – heart failure
IHD – in-hospital death
IVS – interventricular septum
IVCT – isovolumic contraction time
IVRT – isovolumic relaxation time
JVP – jugular venous pressure
LAD – left anterior descending artery
LV – left ventricle
MI – myocardial infarction
MPI – myocardial performance (Tei) index
MRI – magnetic resonance imaging
OR_{adj} – adjusted odds ratio
PA – pulmonary artery
PDA – posterior descending artery
PH – pulmonary hypertension
PHD – post-hospital death
PCI – percutaneous coronary intervention
RCA – right coronary artery

RH – re-hospitalization

RV – right ventricle

RVOT – right ventricle outflow trackt

SA – sino-atrial

STEMI – ST-elevation myocardial infarction

SVT – supraventricular tachyarrhythmia

VA – ventricular arrhythmia

Introduction

Sir William Harvey was the first to describe the importance of right ventricular (RV) function long ago, however, for many years until recently, emphasis was placed on left ventricular (LV) physiology, and little attention has been devoted to RV, because it was considered to have a secondary role in the prognostic evaluation of main cardiac diseases [1-3].

Researchers underestimated RV physiological importance in the maintenance of normal overall hemodynamic performance and described it as just a passive conduit with minimal pumping capability which just connects right atrium (RA) with pulmonary artery (PA) [4]. Such approaches were mainly due the fact that the evaluation of RV function was technically difficult (difficulty in accurately measuring RV volume as a result of its complex geometry etc.).

Since 1990s, advances in echocardiography (EchoCG) and magnetic resonance imaging (MRI) have created new opportunities for the study of RV anatomy and physiology [5, 6]. Importance of RV was recognized after some diagnostic criteria have been introduced to evaluate functions of both ventricles [7]. Since then, the importance of RV function has been recognized in pulmonary hypertension (PH), valvular defects, heart failure (HF), myocardial infarction (MI) [8-10]. Currently, RV is seen as one which has unique anatomical patterns and significant physiological importance [11, 12].

Despite clinical manifestation of right ventricular myocardial infarction (RVMI) was first described by Saunders over 80 years ago as the triad of arterial hypotension (AH), elevated jugular venous pressure, and clear lung fields in a patient with extensive necrosis of the RV and minimal involvement of the left ventricle, as a distinct clinical phenomenon it was recognized only after the report of Cohn in 1974 [13, 14].

Currently RVMI is recognized as an important cardiovascular disease as it defines a significant clinical entity, which is associated with considerable immediate morbidity and mortality and has a well-delineated set of priorities for its management.

Chapter 1. Anatomical and Physiological Characteristics of Right ventricle

Anatomy and physiology of right ventricle

Functional imaging capabilities are improved and it is now well appreciated that there exists some independence between the LV and RV systolic function and diastolic load [15]. Current researchers show an increasing interest in the RV particularly with regard to RV dysfunction and RV HF associated with ST-elevation myocardial infarction (STEMI) with an involvement of the same ventricle [16]. For this reason as well as to escalate investigations in the field of RV physiology, in 2006, the National Heart, Lung, and Blood Institute declared RV physiology as one of priorities in cardiovascular research [16].

RV muscle mass is about one-sixth that of the LV. This could be explained by different loading conditions of ventricles [17]. While the normal LV is thick walled and ellipsoid in shape, the RV is thin walled (3–4 mm) and complex shaped due to the interventricular septum (IVS) [18]. Being an anatomical part of the LV, however, IVS is directed obliquely backward to the right, and curved with the convexity toward the RV [12].

In contrast to the near conical shape of the LV, the RV is more triangular in shape on lateral and semi-lunar on vertical projections. The shape of the RV is partly influenced by the position of the IVS, which curves over the LV during both systole and diastole. In addition, the RV differs from the LV by having strict trabeculae, septomarginal trabecula (or moderator band) and inter-valve fibros tissues [19].

The geometry of the RV is complex. This ventricle consists of an inlet portion and an outlet section separated by the trabecular apex. For some researchers such anatomico-phsysiological description of the RV looks much appropriate than traditional division into two regions (sinus and conus), because apical trabeculae allows distinguishing between morphologically right and left ventricles regardless of location of major mass of ventricle (figure 1). Muscular trabeculae are thicker in the apex of morphological RV while they are smooth and crosswise within the LV [19-21].

Figure 1. Diagram of the right ventricle demonstrating its 3 major chamber components; inflow tract, infundibulum (outflow tract), and apex (Adopted from Kenneth et al., 2009)

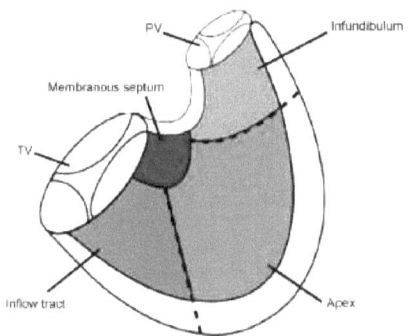

Under normal circumstances, the RV pumps on average the same effective stroke volume as the LV [22]. Interestingly, the LV extracts approximately 75% of the oxygen delivered by coronary blood flow, whereas the RV oxygen extraction is only about 50% under the same rate and stroke volume because of the low resistance of the pulmonary vasculature [16]. Compared with the systemic circulation, pulmonary circulation has a much lower vascular resistance, greater PA distensibility, and a lower peripheral pulse wave reflection coefficient, thus, preventing organs and tissues from congested impairment [23]. In addition, under normal conditions, right-sided pressures are significantly lower than comparable left-sided pressures. RV isovolumic contraction time (IVCT) is shorter because RV systolic pressure rapidly exceeds the low PA diastolic pressure [24].

The IVS and free wall contribute approximately equally to the RV function. The RV free wall is mainly composed of superficial and deep muscle layers [19]. The fibers of the superficial layer are arranged more or less circumferentially in a direction that is parallel to the atrioventricular (AV) groove. The deep muscle fibers of the RV are longitudinally aligned from base to apex. In contrast to the RV, the LV contains obliquely oriented myofibers superficially, longitudinally oriented myofibers in the subendocardium, and predominantly circular fibers in between. This arrangement contributes to the more complex movement of the RV, which includes torsion, translation, rotation, and thickening [19, 23]. In general, longitudinal

7

shortening is a greater contributor to the RV stroke volume than circumferential shortening [24].

The RV contraction is sequential, starting with the contraction of the inlet and trabeculated myocardium and ending with the contraction of the infundibulum (approximately 25 to 50 ms apart). Contraction of the infundibulum is of longer duration than contraction of the inflow region. In general, the RV contracts much in longitudinal rather than radial way [23].

Left-to-right systolic ventricular interaction originates from transmission of systolic forces between the ventricles through the IVS and from the mechanical effect of the common muscle fibers encircling their free walls [26, 27]. Most importantly, any reduction of LV free wall function is immediately translated in a lower RV pressure or function [28-30].

Mutually systolic interaction between the LV and RV mainly works through the IVS yet pericardium has a little role. Rather, the pericardium becomes important in diastolic interaction of two ventricles. Systolic ventricular interaction is more important for RV systolic function, and one-third of the RV potential systolic pressure is generated by the LV [31].

Conversely, the RV pressure overload, as may occur with PH states, may compromise LV function and lead to coincident evidence of LV HF, such as pulmonary edema or effusion. Furthermore, when the RV fails in the setting of LV HF, it may be unable to maintain the flow volume required to maintain adequate LV preload. Because of the multiple influences affecting RV function due to LV HF, RV status may constitute a "common final pathway" in the progression of congestive HF and therefore may be a sensitive indicator of impending decompensation or poor prognosis [32]. In addition, because of the different shape of RV pressure-volume curves, maximal RV elastance better reflects RV contractility than does the end-systolic elastance commonly used in LV pressure-volume interpretation [33].

It is widely accepted that the complex relationship between RV contractility, preload, and afterload can be better understood with the help of pressure-volume loops which depict instantaneous pressure-volume curves under different loading conditions. The slope of the end-systolic pressure-volume relationship is referred to as ventricular elastance which is considered as the most reliable index of contractility [34, 35].

The RV afterload results from a dynamic interplay between resistance, elastance, and wave reflection [36]. In contrary to the LV, the RV demonstrates a higher sensitivity to afterload change [37]. Although in clinical practice, pulmonary vascular resistance is the most commonly used index of afterload, it may not reflect the complex nature of ventricular afterload. Within physiological limits, an increase in the RV preload improves myocardial contraction on the basis of the Frank-Starling mechanism. Beyond the physiological range, excessive RV volume loading can compress the LV and impair global ventricular function through the mechanism of ventricular interdependence [37].

Compared with the LV filling, the RV filling normally starts before and finishes after. The RV isovolumic relaxation time (IVRT) is shorter, and RV filling velocities and the E/A ratio are lower. The respiratory variations in RV filling velocities are, however, more pronounced [38]. Many factors influence RV filling, including intravascular volume status, ventricular relaxation, ventricular chamber compliance, heart rate, passive and active atrial characteristics, LV filling, and pericardial constraint [39].

The RV follows a force-interval relationship in which stroke volume increases above baseline after longer filling periods [33]. In addition, the RV compliance is believed to be greater than the LV compliance [40]. In addition, the pericardium imposes greater constraint on the thinner, more compliant, low-pressure RV [23]. Acute ischemia of the RV is characterized by common shifts in IVCT and partially IVRT [32].

Blood supply of the right ventricle

The right heart has its own unique blood supply system which is a part of the coronary circulation which begins with the coronary arteries arising from the ascending aorta, through openings called coronary ostia which are located above the aortic valves.

There are two main coronary arteries that branch from the ascending aorta, known as the left and right coronary arteries (RCA). In essence, the left main coronary artery supplies the LA, IVS, LV and the anterior wall of the RA. On the other hand, the RCA supplies the RA, the RV as well as the sino-atrial (SA) node [41].

As with the RV, its blood supply is provided not only by the RCA but also by the left anterior descending artery (LAD) and left circumflex (Cx) coronary artery [42]. The RCA arises from the right aortic sinus, running towards the right hand side of the heart, deep to the right auricle and along the right AV groove. From here, it curls around towards the inferior surface of the heart and in 90% of patients forming the posterior interventricular branch at the crux of the heart, more commonly known as the posterior descending artery (PDA) [43]. The distal extent of the RCA varies and may extend posteriorly as far as the obtuse margin of the heart. The PDA runs along the posterior interventiculas sulcus, to supply blood to the walls of the LA and RV, AV node and the posterior aspect of the IVS (figure 2).

Figure 2. Coronary artery system

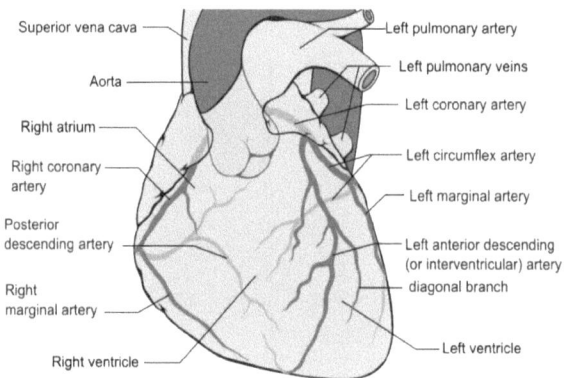

The first branch arising from the RCA is the conal or infundibular branch, which courses anteriorly to supply the muscular right ventricular outflow tract (RVOT) or infundibulum. The RCA supplies blood to the atria with a highly variable pattern of small branches. The sinus node artery arises from the proximal RCA in approximately 50% of patients [44].

The left coronary ostium is usually single, giving rise to a short, common left coronary artery trunk that branches into the LAD and the left Cx arteries. The LAD courses in the anterior interventricular groove, giving rise to the anterior septal perforating branches as it extends toward the cardiac apex. Small branches may arise from the LAD and supply the anterior wall of the RV. Diagonal branches arise from the LAD and course at downward angles to supply the anterolateral free wall of the left ventricle.

The left Cx artery courses along the left AV groove, around the obtuse margin, and posteriorly toward the crux of the heart. Should the Cx reach the crux of the heart and supply the posterior descending coronary artery, the left coronary system would be termed dominant. This occurs in approximately 10% of patients. Atrial branches may arise from the left Cx and supply the sinus node in 40% of patients. Obtuse marginal branches arise from the circumflex system to supply the posterolateral aspect of the LV. In an estimated 70% of patients, a coronary branch (intermedius) arises early off the left coronary system to supply an area between diagonal branches from the LAD and obtuse branches from the circumflex systems.

Before turning towards the diaphragmatic surface of the heart the RCA gives rise to the right marginal branch which runs along the right margin, to supply the wall of the RV. Again, the RCA gives rise to several more branches. Important branches from the RCA include the conus branch and the SA node artery, passing upwards to the aurical wall to the junction between superior vena cava, sulcus termanalis and right auricle.

Variations that occur in less than 1% of the general population may be considered abnormal or anomalies [44]. Most of these variations appear to be of no clinical significance, although a high origin of the ostia may reduce diastolic coronary artery blood flow [45].

The blood supply of the RV varies according to the dominance of the coronary system. In fact, the artery that supplies the PDA determines the coronary dominance. If the PDA is supplied by the RCA, then the coronary circulation can be classified as "right-dominant". If the PDA is supplied by the Cx artery, a branch of the left artery, then the coronary circulation can be classified as "left-dominant". If the PDA is supplied by both the RCA and the Cx, then the coronary circulation can be classified as "co-dominant" [46].

In the segmentar model of coronary system, right dominancy assumes the RCA dominancy for segments from 1 to 9, while left dominancy is provided by the left coronary artery and involves segments of 18-19th and 23-27th [46].

In a right-dominant system, which is found in ≈80% of the population, the RCA supplies most of the RV [23, 42]. The lateral wall of the RV is supplied by the marginal branches of the RV, whereas the posterior wall and the inferoseptal region are supplied by the PDA. The anterior wall of the RV and the anteroseptal region are supplied by branches of the left anterior descending artery. The infundibulum derives its supply from the conal artery, which has a separate ostial origin in 30% of cases. The separate ostium explains the preservation of infundibular contraction in the presence of proximal right coronary occlusion [23, 42].

In the absence of severe RV hypertrophy or pressure overload, proximal RCA flow occurs during both systole and diastole [43]. However, beyond the RV marginal branches, diastolic coronary blood flow predominates. The relative resistance of the RV to irreversible ischemic injury may be explained by its lower oxygen consumption, its more extensive collateral system, especially from the moderator band artery, a branch of the first septal perforator that originates from the left anterior descending coronary artery, and its ability to increase oxygen extraction [47].

Chapter 2. Right Ventricular Myocardial Infarction: Pathopsysiology, Epidemiology, Diagnostics, Clinical characteristics and Treatment

Interestingly, RVMI noted at necropsy usually involves the posterior septum and posterior wall rather than the right free wall. The relative sparing of the right ventricular anterior wall apparently arises from a high degree of collateralization. This collateral blood flow is thought to be derived from the thebesian veins and diffusion of oxygen directly from the ventricular cavity.

A direct correlation exists between the anatomic site of the RCA occlusion and the extent of RVMI. Studies have demonstrated that more proximal RCA occlusions result in larger RVMI [48, 49]. On occasion, the RV can be subjected to infarction from occlusion of the Cx artery [50].

Because the RV is considered a low-pressure volume pump, its contractility is highly dependent on diastolic pressure. Hence, when contractility and associated diastolic dysfunction are impaired attendant to RVMI, the RV diastolic pressure increases substantially and systolic pressure decreases. In such circumstances, concomitant LV dysfunction, with increase in RV afterload, is possible. In such a setting, RV output can decrease dramatically, and the only driving force remaining is elevated RA pressure. In such a circumstance, the RV serves as a poorly functioning conduit between the RA and the PA [51].

Elevation of the RA pressure secondary to RVMI has been noted to serve as a stimulus for secretion of atrial natriuretic factor. Increased levels of this polypeptide can be detrimental to normal left ventricular filling pressures. This occurs by virtue of the potent vasodilating, natriuretic, diuretic, and aldosterone-inhibiting properties of atrial natriuretic factor. Inappropriately elevated levels of atrial natriuretic factor may worsen the clinical syndrome of RVMI [52]. The potential hemodynamic derangements associated with RVMI render the afflicted patient unusually sensitive to diminished preload (ie, volume) and loss of AV synchrony. These two circumstances can result in a severe decrease in right and, secondarily, left, ventricular output [53].

Acute MI involving only the RV is a rare event, yet RV-involvement in the setting of acute inferior wall myocardial infarctions (STEMI) is much more frequent [54]. Acute occlusion of the RCA, proximal to the right ventricular branches, results in right ventricular dysfunction, however, many right coronary artery occlusions do not result in significant right ventricular necrosis [55].

Early thrombolysis or mechanical reperfusion of an occluded coronary artery resulting in RVMI is associated with prompt reduction in RA pressure. This is extremely important because persistently elevated RA pressure has been associated with increased in-hospital mortality when associated with MI.

The extent of RVMI varies greatly and is dependent on the site of occlusion of the right ventricular arterial supply. If occlusion occurs before the right ventricular marginal branches and if collateral blood flow from the LAD is absent, then the size of infarction generally is greater. Extent of infarction depends somewhat on flow through the thebesian veins [56, 57].

In general, any major reduction in blood supply to the right ventricular free wall portends an adverse prognosis in association with this disorder. Total occlusion of the RCA typically manifests as ST-segment elevation in the inferior leads and sometimes the lateral precordial leads of the surface electrocardiogram (ECG).

Epidemiology of Right Ventricular Myocardial Infarction

Historically, the incidence of RVMI depends on the criteria used for detection. Early autopsy studies suggested that RVMI accompanies fatal STEMI 24-34% of cases [58, 59]. Noninvasive studies suggest that RVMI occurs in more than 30% of patients with acute inferior-posterior LV MI [60, 61].

Isolated RVMI is extremely rare; it is usually noted in association with STEMI. The incidence of RVMI in such cases ranges from 10-50%, depending on the series [62].

The frequency of RVMI, which can be detected by right-sided precordial leads, in association with non-ST-segment elevation or non-Q-wave MI, is not known and currently is being investigated. Although RVMI is clinically evident in a sizable number of cases, the incidence is considerably less than that found at autopsy [54, 63, 64]. A major reason for the discrepancy is the difficulty in establishing the presence of the RVMI in living subjects. Additionally, RV dysfunction and stunning frequently are of a transient nature, such that estimation of its true incidence is even more difficult [61, 64].

Although there are potentially life-threatening acute hemodynamic and clinical consequences in some, most patients with RV dysfunction after MI have spontaneous recovery of RV function, leading some clinicians to believe that the term "right ventricular infarction" is a misnomer and represents viable but "stunned" myocardium [65].

Criteria have been set forth to diagnose RVMI; even when strictly employed, however, the criteria lead to underestimation of the true incidence of RVMI [66].

Pathophysiology and clinical presentation of Right Ventricular Myocardial Infarction

Clinical recognition of acute RVMI is extremely important, as appropriate therapy for hypotension and cardiogenic shock (CS) must be started prior to consideration of noninvasive tests or invasive monitoring. The RVMI should be suspected in any patient with acute STEMI.

Ischemia or infarction of the RV results in decreased right ventricular compliance, reduced filling, and decreased RV stroke volume. These changes lead to diminished LV filling and drop in cardiac output. In addition, acute right ventricular dilatation causes a leftward shift of IVS, increasing left ventricular end-diastolic pressure with a decrease of left ventricular compliance and cardiac output [67].

These changes in left ventricular compliance are further aggravated by increased intrapericardial pressure as a result of right ventricular dilatation [68]. Brookes et al. demonstrated that the geometric changes in the LV, caused by right ventricular dilatation due to RVMI, resulted in a significant impairment of left ventricular contractile function in addition to the diastolic filling abnormalities and changes in compliance [69]. Therefore, although the patient has clinical signs of increased right-sided pressure, the LV filling and systolic function may be below normal.

The symptoms of RVMI may be more pronounced in the presence of combined RA infarction with associated rate and rhythm disturbances [55]. When the culprit coronary artery lesion is distal to the right atrial branches, augmented RA contractility enhances RV performance and offsets some of the hemodynamic consequences of RVMI.

The triad of hypotension, elevated jugular venous pressure (JVP), and clear lung fields has been recognized as marker of RVMI in acute STEMI [14, 70].

The reason for the development of hypotension in patients with RV involvement during STEMI may be due to reduction of stroke volume of RV or association with activation of vagus system. Hypotension is eligibly more frequent in RVMI patients than those inferior MI patients without RV involvement [71]. RVMI ranges in its hemodynamic features from a normotensive state to a severe CS state that is resistant to any treatment. Also, concomitant LV infarction affects the hemodynamic outcome associated with RVMI.

According to Shock Registry Data, patients with predominant RV shock were younger than patients with LV shock, although coronary artery disease risk factor profile, with the exception of hyperlipidemia, was similar between the two groups. There was a lower incidence of previous MI for patients with predominant RV shock, although the prevalence of other comorbid conditions such as renal insufficiency, peripheral vascular disease, and previous revascularization was similar to that in patients with LV shock [72].

The severity of the hemodynamic abnormalities associated with RVMI is related to the extent of RV ischemia and consequent RV dysfunction as well as to the restraining effect of the pericardium, LV function, and ventricular interdependence [73]. The intact LV may assist RV ejection by LV septal contraction causing a bulging into the RV which generates an active RV systolic pressure wave and systolic force sufficient for pulmonary perfusion. Loss of this mechanism with concomitant LV infarction, particularly when the IVS is involved, may lead to further hemodynamic deterioration in patients with RVMI. Furthermore, augmented atrial contraction is necessary to overcome the stiffness of the ischemic RV, and factors that impair RV filling (intravascular volume depletion, concomitant atrial infarction, and loss of AV synchrony) may severely compromise hemodynamics and result in CS. It is consistent with the systemic hypotension and LV dysfunction that occurs even when RVMI is responsible for shock and supports previous reports noting that the hemodynamic consequence of RV dysfunction is the result of a critical interaction between both ventricles with the IVS shift into the LV [74].

In comparison to the LV, the RV is poorly adapted to compensate for the increase in afterload, with its large surface area and thin free wall, and this may explain the rapid hemodynamic compromise and earlier onset of hypotension and shock in patients with predominant RV shock [75]. In these patients, the RA pressure is elevated with either normal or slightly elevated pulmonary capillary wedge pressure. If the RVMI is extensive, the RA and RV tressure wave forms may be identical suggesting absence of any effective RV contraction. Cardiac output and cardiac index would be expected to be similar for patients with predominant RV or LV shock once shock ensues.

The higher number of cases with JVP prominence in patients with RV involvement may be due to increasing of end diastolic pressure of right ventricle in

RVMI. Pulsus paradoxus (decrease in size, or even momentary disappearance of the pulse during inspiration) and Kussmaul's sign (an inspiratory increase in JVP) have also been reported in patients with have also been reported in patients with RVMI [70]. The presence of elevated JVP and Kussmaul's sign in the setting of an acute STEMI indicate a hemodynamically significant RVI35 (sensitivity - 88% and specificity - 100%), particularly when it is associated with significant damage to the LV and/or IVS [76]. In some cases, these symptoms are not present at admission and do not occur until diuretics or nitrates are administered.

Auscultation may reveal a right-sided S3 and S4. Tricuspid regurgitation may be identified because of dilatation of right ventricular chamber, which may be severe when related to papillary muscle dysfunction [77].

Finally, high-grade AV blocks and other arrhythmias may occur and result in loss of atrial ventricular synchrony with exacerbation of hypotension and shock [78, 79]. Our data suggests that RVMI is associated with higher rates of ≥ Lown III grades ventricular arrhythmia (VA), II-III^{0}AV and/or sino-atrial (SA) heart blocks (HB), supraventricular tachyarrhythmia (SVT), CS, pericarditis (PC) and successful reanimation cases (SRC) [80].

Diagnostics of Right Ventricular Myocardial Infarction

Electrocardiography

In clinical settings, RVMI is often diagnosed by the right pre-cordial electrocardiography (ECG). ECG is recognized as the most simple and readily available diagnostic tool for identification of RVMI.

Because RVMIs are usually associated with an STEMI, evaluation using standard 12-lead ECG often reveals corresponding ST elevations in leads II, III and aVF (figure 3). Disproportionate ST segment elevation with greater ST elevation in lead III than in lead II is pathognomonic for an RVMI [81].

Because standard 12-lead ECG images mainly assess the LV, right-sided precordial leads should always be used. These can show ST segment elevation across the entire right precordium from V_{1R} through V_{6R}; a sole ST segment elevation in lead V_{4R} >1.0 mm is a reliable marker of an RVMI, with 100% sensitivity, 87% specificity and 92% predictive accuracy (figure 4) [82, 83].

Furthermore, higher ST segment elevations in V4R have been found to be independent predictive factors for more significant RV dysfunction and higher

17

mortality rates [84, 85]. This ST-segment elevation is thought to represent an ischemic injury of the posterobasal septum, since this area of contiguous myocardium is invariably damaged in patients who have pathological evidence of STEMI involving the RV [86].

Figure 3. Standard 12-lead ECG of a patient with an inferior STEMI with RVMI

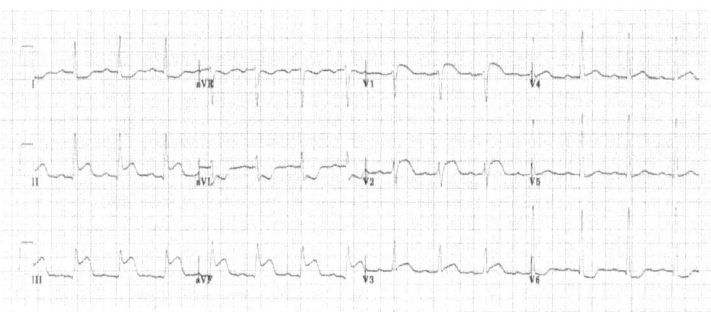

Note: Right ventricular infarction in this patient with inferior STEMI is suggested by ST elevation in V_1 and ST elevation in lead III > lead II.

Figure 4. Right-sided ECG of a patient with an inferior STEMI with RVMI

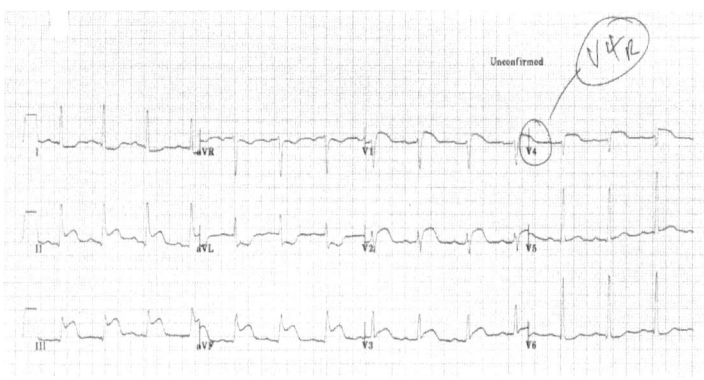

Note: ECG of the same patient with V_{4R} electrode position. There is ST elevation in V_{4R} consistent with RVMI.

18

Thus, ECG serves as a very important tool for the diagnosis of RVMI, and it is imperative to record right-sided precordial leads in all patients with STEMI as soon as possible.

Hemodynamic examination

Hemodynamic examination using right-sided cardiac catheterization may reveal a disproportionate elevation of right-sided filling pressures compared with left-sided filling pressures. The generally accepted criteria for hemodynamically significant RVMIs include RA pressure >10 mmHg, a RA pressure to pulmonary capillary wedge pressure ratio >0.8, or RA pressure within 5 mmHg of the pulmonary capillary wedge pressure ratio. However, with concomitant and significant LV dysfunction, the close relationship between the above two parameters is not preserved, although the RA pressure will continue to be elevated [60, 87].

Echocardiography

Two-dimensional (2D) EchoCG is today a well-established cardiac investigation worldwide. EchoCG has its unique role in the diagnosis of RVMI. Abnormal EchoCG findings include right ventricular dilatation, its wall akinesis or dyskinesis right after some minutes of myocardial necrosis, reversed septal curvature caused by the reversal of the transseptal pressure due to increased right ventricular end-diastolic pressure, and the presence of severe right atrial enlargement (figure 5) [88]. The presence of interatrial septal bowing indicating a concomitant RA infarction is an important marker predicting more hypotension, AV blocks, and higher mortality [89].

Two-dimensional guided M-mode measurements of systolic long axis motion of the RV free wall is an attractive tool due to its simplicity and has been shown to correlate with ejection fraction (EF) derived by radionuclide angiography [91]. It has also been shown to be valuable in assessing ischemic heart disease and cardiomyopathy [92]. The main limitation in assessing RV function using the long axis motion is that it only represents the inflow free wall segments, thus missing the RVOT and the septal contribution to the overall function of the RV.

Figure 5. Right ventricular myocardial infarction (Adopted from D'Arcy Nanda, 1982)

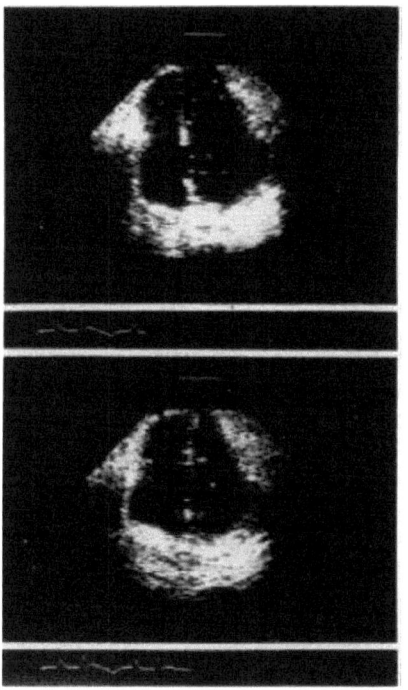

Note: The transducer was placed at the apex and angled inferiorly to view the basal portion of the RV free wall, which demonstrates dyskinesis (upper image taken in diastole; lower image – in systole).

Additional measurements of RVOT fractional shortening add great value. This method has been found to correlate better with PA systolic pressure compared to long axis motion [93]. Finally, RV end-diastolic diameter from the parasternal projection can easily be used as a measurement of dimension [94]. However, as the RV is positioned close to the sternum and being complex in its geometrical shape, assessment by 2D EchoCG may be limited [95].

Volume and EF calculations using Simpson's formula are based on mathematical assumptions of RV geometry, therefore subject to inaccuracies and not useful in clinical practice. RV end-diastolic and end-systolic areas and the calculated fractional area change (FAC) including the trabeculated apical part reflect global and regional wall motion and can be measured both manually and with automatic edge detection

[95]. The McConnell sign, i.e. basal and mid segmental RV hypokinesia with preserved apical wall motion, has been reported in patients with pulmonary embolism and those with RVMI [96]. Finally, RA area can easily be measured from the apical four-chamber view. From the subcostal view, evaluation of pericardial effusion and its involvement with RV free wall function can be achieved. Additional estimation of RA pressure can be obtained from measuring the inferior vena cava dimensions and its diameter variation during normal breathing or sniff test. A reduction in inferior vena cava diameter of more than 50% is consistent with right atrial pressure <10 mmHg [97].

Standard 2D EchoCG of the RV usually includes a set of standardized views to differentiate normal RV structure and function from abnormal and to assess RV size, volume, and contractility. These include parasternal long-axis, parasternal RV inflow, PSAX, apical 4-chamber, RV-focused apical 4-chamber, and subcostal views (table 1) [98].

Table 1. Main echocardiographic views of assessment of the right ventricle

Echocardiographic views	Suggested measurments
Parasternal long-axis view	RVOT end-diastolic dimenstion
Parasternal long-axis view of RV inflow (modified long-axis view)	Anatint and function of tricuspid valve (anterior and posterior leaflets)
RVOT	Pulmonary valve
Short-axis parasternal views at different levels	RVOT end-systolic and end-diastolic dimenstions
	RVOT shortening fraction
	LV eccentricity index
Apical 4-chamber view	RV dimentions at long and short axises
	TAPSE
	FAC
	Tricuspidal valve (anterior and posterior leaflets)
Subcostal views (4-chamber and short-axis)	RV free wall tickness

A Doppler examination of specific pulmonary regurgitation patterns can add hemodynamic insight and confirm the diagnosis of RV involvement, especially in cases of technically inadequate two-dimensional images [99].

Standard 2D EchoCG provides images for the comprehensive assessment of RV systolic and diastolic function. A number of methods have been proposed for the quantitative EchoCG assessment of global RV function although none has achieved widespread clinical use. As for RV systolic function, more studies have demonstrated the clinical utility and value of FAC, tricuspid annular plane systolic excursion (TAPSE), myocardial performance index (MPI) and S' of the tricuspid annulus.

FAC is easily obtained using the apical four-chamber view in wich the end-diastolic and end-systolic areas are simply planimetered. FAC is obtained by tracing the RV endocardium both in systole and diastole from the annulus, along the free wall to the apex, and then back to the annulus, along the IVS (figure 6).

Figure 6. EchoCG measurment of RV FAC

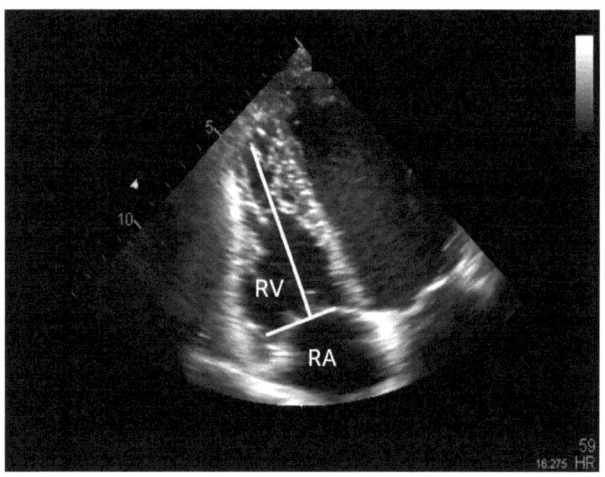

The FAC (as a percentage) is expressed as:

$$FAC\ (\%) = \frac{(End - Diastoloc\ Area) - (End - Systolic\ Area)}{(End - Diastoloc\ Area)}$$

According to the recommendations of the American Society of Echocardiography normal values are greater than 35% [98]. It is a measure of RV systolic function that has been shown to correlate with RV EF by MRI. RV FAC was found to be an independent predictor of HF, sudden death, stroke, and/or mortality in studies of patients after MI [100, 101].

TAPSE: The systolic movement of the base of the RV free wall provides one of the most visibly obvious movements on normal EchoCG. TAPSE is a method to measure the distance of systolic excursion of the RV annular segment along its longitudinal plane, from a standard apical 4-chamber window. TAPSE represents longitudinal function of the right ventricle in the same way as mitral annular plane systolic excursion by Doppler tissue imaging does with the left ventricle.

It is inferred that the greater the descent of the base in systole, the better the RV systolic function. As with other regional methods, it assumes that the displacement of the basal and adjacent segments in the apical 4-chamber view is representative of the function of the entire right ventricle, an assumption that is not valid in many disease states or when there are regional RV wall motion abnormalities. TAPSE is usually acquired by placing an M-mode cursor through the tricuspid annulus and measuring the amount of longitudinal motion of the annulus at peak systole.

In the initial validation study by Kaul et al, TAPSE correlated strongly with radionuclide angiography, with low interobserver variability [102]. A TAPSE cutoff value < 17 mm yielded high specificity, though low sensitivity to distinguish abnormal from normal subjects [103].

TAPSE is simple, less dependent on optimal image quality, and reproducible, and it does not require sophisticated equipment or prolonged image analysis. However, TAPSE assumes that the displacement of a single segment represents the function of a complex 3D structure. Furthermore, it is angle dependent, and there are no large-scale validation studies. Finally, TAPSE may be load dependent.

The **MPI**, also known as **Tei index**, is a global estimate of both systolic and diastolic function of the RV. It is based on the relationship between ejection and non-ejection work of the heart. The MPI is defined as the ratio of isovolumic time divided by ejection time (ET) [104].

The MPI is expressed as:

$$MPI = \frac{(\text{Isovolumic relaxation time}) + (\text{Isovolumic contriction time})}{(\text{Ejection time})}$$

The measure remains accurate within a broad range of heart rates, though the components should be measured with a constant R-R interval to minimize error [105]. Although the MPI was initially thought to be relatively independent of preload, this has been questioned in more recent studies. In addition, the MPI has been demonstrated to be unreliable when RA pressure is elevated (eg, RVMI), as there is a more rapid equilibration of pressures between the RV and RA, shortening the IVRT and resulting in an inappropriately small MPI [106].

The right-sided MPI can be obtained by two methods: the pulsed Doppler method and the tissue Doppler method. In the pulsed Doppler method, the ET is measured with pulsed Doppler of RV outflow (time from the onset to the cessation of flow), and the tricuspid (valve) closure-opening time is measured with either pulsed Doppler of the tricuspid inflow (time from the end of the transtricuspid A wave to the beginning of the transtricuspid E wave) or continuous Doppler of the TR jet (time from the onset to the cessation of the jet). These measurements are taken from different images, and one must therefore attempt to use beats with similar R-R intervals to obtain a more accurate RV MPI value.

In the tissue Doppler method, all time intervals are measured from a single beat by pulsing the tricuspid annulus. As was demonstrated for the LV MPI, it is important to note that the correlation between both methods is modest and that normal values differ on the basis of the method chosen [107].

The MPI has prognostic value in patients with PH at a single point in time, and changes in MPI correlate with change in clinical status in this patient group [107, 108]. It has also been studied in RVMI, hypertrophic cardiomyopathy, and congenital heart disease, among others [109, 110].

Several studies have recently shown that LV MPI has a prognostic value for clinical outcomes in MIs and many authors underlined usefulness of this index for practical implementation, especially, for risk stratification purposes [111]. Particularly, LV MPI has been shown to be a useful, sensitive, and reproducible indicator for myocardial dysfunction in many clinical settings in distinguishing patients with a poor in-hospital outcome, and its value as an independent predictor of cardiac events during hospitalization [112-114]. Also, it has been demonstrated that LV MPI predicts LV remodeling [115] and improvement of LV MPI closely reflects intrinsic improvement of cardiac function [116]. Further, in late phase of AMI the index has shown prognostic value regarding death, HF, and new cardiac events [117, 118].

The upper reference limit is 0.40 by pulsed Doppler and 0.55 by tissue Doppler. This approach is feasible in a large majority of subjects both with and without tricuspid regurgitation, the MPI is reproducible, and it avoids the geometric assumptions and limitations of complex RV geometry. The pulsed tissue Doppler method allows for measurement of MPI as well as S', E', and A', all from a single image. However, The MPI is unreliable when RV ET and TR time are measured with differing R-R intervals, as in atrial fibrillation. Moreover, it is load dependent and unreliable when RA pressure is elevated.

Radionuclide ventriculography and 99mTc pyrophosphate myocardial scintigraphy

A 99mTc pyrophosphate myocardial scintigraphy examination requires proper timing, and the scans are usually not diagnostic until 72 hours after the onset of symptoms. Excessive uptake of the radionuclide in non-cardiac structures (chest wall, bone, cartilage) can lead to issues regarding the interpretation of the acquired images [87]. A dilated RV with hypokinesia, akinesia or dyskinesia of its free wall associated with a depressed RV EF and a normal or only mildly depressed LV EF are indicative of an RVMI [61].

Cardiac magnetic resonance (CMR)

CMR using late gadolinium enhancement imaging enables the accurate characterization of ischaemic myocardial injury. CMR studies have indicated that RVMI occurs in a high number of cases in patients with STEMI (47-57%) and that some patients with anterior MI (11-65%) also have RV involvement to some extent [75]. Indeed, two observational reports comparing the frequency of RV involvement between different modalities in patients with acute MI indicated that RV involvement was detected significantly more frequently with CMR than with ECG or EchoCG [119, 120]. Although the recent advances in CMR may contribute to understanding the pathology as well as providing a more accurate diagnosis of RVMI, further investigations are essential to establish the usefulness of the CMR technique, since the numbers of patients included in these observational studies were limited.

Therapy of Right Ventricular Myocardial Infarction

RV ischemia may lead to systolic and diastolic dysfunction, resulting in a serious deficit in LV preload with a subsequent drop in cardiac output and consequent systemic hypotension. Adequate filling (preload) of the impaired RV is thus crucial to maintain sufficient RV output volume and LV function [67]. Fluid replacement can be challenging in some patients with RVMI, particularly in the presence of severe RV dysfunction [121]. Therefore, the initial therapy for hypotension in patients with RVMI without pulmonary congestion has traditionally been volume expansion, particularly if the estimated central venous pressure was <15 mmHg at the same time, it is critically important to avoid drugs that cause venodilation and a decrease in RV filling (eg, nitrates, diuretics) [122]. In previous studies, maintenance of the RV preload with volume loading and normal saline alone was thought to resolve the accompanying hypotension and improve the cardiac output [43]. The typical regimen consisted of normal saline (40 ml/min, up to total of 2 l, intravenously), while maintaining the right atrial pressure (RAP) at <18 mmHg to prevent volume overload [123]. Some authors recommended beginning with a volume challenge of 300 mL to 600 mL normal saline over 10 min to 15 min through a central line or through a large-bore peripheral intravenous site [124]. However, later clinical studies reported variable responses to aggressive fluid therapy with a target pulmonary wedge pressure (PWP) of 18–24 mmHg [61, 125]. Some studies have indicated that volume loading may not increase cardiac output [61, 68, 125]. This may be due to variable initial volume status among patients.

Some patients may be relatively volume-depleted and could benefit from a volume infusion, while others who present with a normal intravascular volume show no changes in cardiac index or blood pressure following a fluid load because the RV preload is already at a maximum for maintaining RV stroke output [87]. Some studies showed that volume loading further elevates the right-sided filling pressure without improving cardiac output [68, 125, 126]. Berisha and associates reported that the maximal RV stroke work index occurred when the filling pressure was 10–14 mmHg, and a mean RAP of >14 mmHg was almost always associated with a reduced RV stroke work index [127]. Although the hemodynamic characteristics of RVMI may be extremely variable, depending on the patient's state of hydration and the degree of concomitant LV involvement, this study indicated that the mean optimal pulmonary wedge pressure, which corresponded to the maximum LV stroke work index in each patient, was 16 mm Hg. Based on hemodynamic monitoring studies, exceeding a RAP or PCWP of 20 mmHg is generally not recommended [128].

Invasive hemodynamic monitoring is, therefore, recommended, because further infusion may be harmful if additional increases in RV volume prevent sufficient LV filling via inter-ventricular interactions and intrapericardial pressure equalization. If initial volume loading fails to improve arterial pressure and cardiac output despite significant increases in RA pressure and pulmonary capillary wedge pressure, then positive inotropic agent therapy can be effective in stabilizing patients. Dell'Italia et al. studied the effect of dobutamine in patients with RVMI after volume loading and concluded that dobutamine produced a statistically significant increase in cardiac index, stroke volume index and RV EF [128].

Restoration of sufficient coronary blood flow represents the only treatment that addresses the underlying problem, and early reperfusion improves RV performance as well as the clinical course and survival [129]. Because of the higher reperfusion rate achieved with primary angioplasty, the mortality among patients treated with this method has been relatively low.

Our recent study shows that primary percutaneous coronary intervention (PCI) has measurable advantages over standard (non-invasive) treatment approaches in significantly reducing risks of cardiac events both in-hospital and 1-year post-infarction periods in patients with RVMI. Particularly, our data suggests that primary PCI reduces the in-hospital death (IHD) risk by 9.3 times, early post-infarction angina (EPA) risk – by 3.3, VA risk – by 1.6 and CS risk – by 3.0 times, all for in-hospital period. Moreover, primary PCI reduces risks of 1-year post-hospital death (PHD) and re-hospitalization (RH) rates by 4.3 and 3.2 times correspondingly [130, 131].

Asalli et al. reported that complete revascularization of the RCA, including the major RV branch, was more closely associated with a higher recovery rate of RV function by EchoCG and better 30-day mortality than incomplete revascularization in patients with RVMI [132]. Early reperfusion leads to prompt improvement and subsequent recovery of RV free wall contraction and global RV function without any scar formation.

In patients with refractory hypotension and low cardiac output, intra-aortic balloon counterpulsation IABC may be beneficial. Although it does not directly influence RV performance, it can increase coronary perfusion pressure and thereby improve RV function, particularly if the RCA has been recanalized [129].

The limitations of medical management of RV HF have led to the development of a number of RV assist devices designed to bypass the impaired RV and/or pulmonary circulation to allow the right ventricle to recover. The Tandem Heart Percutaneous Ventricular Assist Device (CardiacAssist Inc, USA) is an extracorporeal centrifugal pump that generates continuous flow with a minimal low amplitude pulsatile component. It can provide flow up to 5.0 L/min and pumps the blood from the right atrium to the main pulmonary artery, bypassing a poorly functioning RV. Kapur et al studied nine patients with medically refractory RV HF and found that, although four patients died early, the Percutaneous Ventricular Assist Device was associated with significantly improved hemodynamics [130].

Venoarterial extra-corporeal membrane oxygenation systems can provide both cardiac and respiratory support. These can be fully established through the cannulation of a femoral vein and artery using the Seldinger technique; therefore, surgery is not required. In contrast to RV assist devices, this technique allows total bypassing of the pulmonary bed and, therefore, does not cause further elevation of the pulmonary pressures and relieves the RV overload. Particularly in patients presenting with an obstructive hemodynamic pattern (PH, pulmonary embolism), extracorporeal membrane oxygenation method may be considered to be the only reasonable approach [131, 132].

Prognosis of Right Ventricular Myocardial Infarction

Patients with acute STEMI have a significantly increased risk of death during hospitalization if RV involvement is present. In a meta-analysis, the mortality rate was noted to be higher in the presence of RVMI than in its absence (17% vs. 6.3%), thereby corresponding to an overall relative risk mortality increase of 2.6 [133].

The worse outcome is believed to be attributable to the high incidence of refractory CS as infarcted RV tissue fails to offer a sufficient preload, which will lead to inadequate LV performance and, consequently, a low cardiac output will lead to systemic hypoperfusion. The revascularization strategy has improved the overall short-term mortality rate of acute MI (7% vs. 9%) compared with that associated with the fibrinolytic strategy [134].

However, although the number of patients with RVMI is small, these patients seem to have a higher risk of in-hospital mortality in the mechanical reperfusion era than during the fibrinolytic era. For example, Zehender et al. suggested RV involvement during acute STEMI as a strong, independent predictor of major acute cardiac complications (ACCs) - ventricular tachycardia, ventricular fibrillation, myocardial rupture, II and III^0 AV block requiring cardiac pacing, re-infarction and CS, and in-hospital mortality in patients with acute STEMIs. They also recommended that ECG assessment of RVMI should be routinely performed in all patients with acute STEMIs [84]. In addition, Khan et al. calculated higher in-hospital mortality

(23.5%) as well as other major ACCs in patients with RVMI than those with isolated STEMI (18.1%). They concluded that RVMI is associated with considerable morbidity and mortality, and its presence defines a higher risk subgroup of patients with STEMIs [137]. In another study, Miszalski-Jamka et al. reported that the extent of RVMI and RV dysfunction assessed early after STEMI are independent outcome predictors, which provide incremental prognostic value to clinical data, LV systolic function, and infarct burden [138]. In addition, Kukla et al. in their study showed that RVMI is associated with worse prognosis and increased number of in-hospital ACCs, older patients aged >70 years have definitely poorer prognosis and thrombolytic therapy in a subgroup of older patients with RVI remains ineffective [139]. Despite the advances in therapeutic strategy, including mechanical reperfusion for acute MI, improvement in the in-hospital mortality could not be achieved even by mechanical reperfusion in patients with fatal RVMI, and therefore, the relative risk of in-hospital mortality in such a population might have been highlighted.

The prognosis associated with RVMI is worse in the short term, but those patients who survive hospitalization have a relatively good long-term prognosis [140]. This is in concordance with the findings in patients with LV CS; in the SHOCK study, 1 year after revascularization, the survival curves remained relatively stable with an annual mortality rate of 8-10 deaths per 100 patient-years. This annual mortality rate is comparable to that reported in a broad cohort of post-PCI patients [141]. In addition, Mendes et al. showed that in patients with CS secondary to predominant LV HF, the presence of RV dilatation and dysfunction identifies a subgroup of patients with predominant STEMI and an improved long-term prognosis [142].

However, up to now, data on prognostic role of RV involvement in LV inferior wall MI remains controversial. For example, RV involvement significantly increases mortality in patients with STEMIs, although it does not achieve the same rates observed in anterior wall LVMIs [143]. In their recently published research Foussas et al. found no significant difference in long-term 3-month mortality between patients with and without a RVMI [144]. In another study, Jim et al. found no influence of RV involvement in the prognosis of STEMIs, yet they found advanced age, female gender, lateral wall extension, complete AV block, bundle branch block and cardiac free-wall rupture as independent predictors of poor in-hospital outcome in the same patients [145]. Some authors assume that a real prognostic role has the size of myocardial necrosis or life-threatening arrhythmias rather than the presence of RVMI [143, 146].

Our recent prospective study confirmed early negative and long-term (1-year) positive predictive importance of RV involvement in 596 consecutive patients (85.9% males, mean age: 57.3) with primary STEMI admitted to the Department of Urgent Cardiology of Erebouni MC, Yerevan, Armenia [147, 148]. The study population was categorized into 2 groups: non-RVMI (n=338) and RVMI (n=258). After the MI all pts were followed 1 year.

We compared STEMI patients with and without RV involvement and calculated adjusted to all major covariates (age, gender, and accompanying diseases like Diabetes Miletus (DM), AH, and chronic obstructive pulmonary diseases' (COPD) odds ratios (OR_{adj}) for main in-hospital and post-infarction outcomes (table 2).

In addition, we found a significant difference in surveillances between the above groups for the combined post-infarction death and rehospitalization events (figure 7).

Table 2. A summary of early and 1-year predictive pattern of RV involvement in patients with STEMI

Clinical outputs	No RVIM group (% ± SD)	RVIM group (% ± SD)	OR_{adj}	P value
In-hospital cardiac death	3.8±3.5%	10.5±49%	3.0	p<0.002
Early post-infarction angina	25.7±8.0%	24.8±6.9%	-	Not significant
Ventricular extrasystoly ≥ Lown III°	16.9±6.9%	33.3±7.6%	2.5	p<0.001
II-III° SA or AV HB	11.8±5.9%	33.3±7.6%	3.8	p<0.001
Supraventricular tachyarrhythmia	3.8±3.5%	17.8±6.1%	5.1	p<0.001
Cardiogenic shock	2.7±2.4%	13.2±5.4%	5.7	p<0.001
Pericarditis	3.3±3.0%	11.2±5.1%	3.6	p<0.001
Successful reanimation cases	4.1±3.7%	10.9±5.0%	2.6	p<0.005
Life-threatening ACCs (VA or II-III^0 AV or SA HB or CS or SRC)	32,5±5,8%	67,1±7,5%	4.2	p<0.001
Post-infarction cardiac death	11.9±5.6%	6.0±3.5%	2.5	p<0.009
Re-hospitalization	18.9±6.8%	11.2±4.6%	2.0	p<0.007

Figure 7. Logistic survival curves for complex endpoint of post-infarction death and/or rehospitalization cases in patients with or without RV involvement STEMI

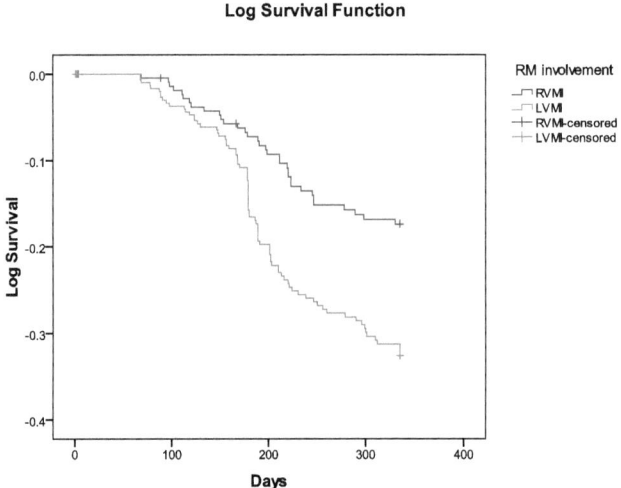

Conclusion

RVMI often accompanies an STEMI presenting with typical clinical, ECG and EchoCG findings. In the presence of hypotension or CS without signs of LV HF and 1 mm ST segment elevation in the V_{4R} lead, a diagnosis of RVMI is highly probable. Specific treatment includes fluid loading and vasopressors, which should be administered immediately. In addition, patients with RV involvement require continuous careful monitoring because they are at a significantly higher risk for ventricular fibrillation, sustained ventricular tachycardia and high-degree AV blocks, any of which would worsen the in-hospital prognosis. RVMI appears to have positive long-term prognosis.

Chapter 3. Prognostic Value of Echocardiographic Parameters in Patients with Inferior STEMI

In this chapter we will present key results of our study on assessment of predictive patterns of traditional EchoCG parameters as well as suggested combinations of the same measurements in patients with primary STEMI.

The Study Rationale

As it was discussed earlier, clinical outcomes of patients after MI are determined by the interaction of a large number of factors. Besides the importance of clinical parameters, recent studies demonstrated the usefulness of standard 2D EchoCG and Doppler myocardial imaging (DMI) for identification of patients who are at risk of adverse outcome [54]. It was revealed that the presence of LV dysfunction on EchoCG shortly after MI is one of the most important prognostic parameters indicating worse long-term outcomes [117]. From Doppler criteria, LV MPI - a numeric value obtained by using cardiac time intervals - is currently accepted as a useful global estimator of both systolic and diastolic myocardial function of LV [104, 105].

The relevance of RV function, on the other hand, is poorly defined in MI patients [149]. However, involvement of the RV during STEMI has been recently defined by several authors as a strong predictor of hospital mortality [84, 150, 151].

Currently, TAPSE - a distance of systolic excursion of the RV annular segment along its longitudinal plane from a standard apical 4-chamber window - is widely recognized as a clinically useful and feasible marker of RV dysfunction, and has been proven to be a valuable prognostic estimator in various cardiac diseases [152].

However, data on practical usefulness of standard 2D echocardiography and DMI parameters in patients with primary STEMI so that RV could be involved in infarction and lead to RV dysfunction is lacking. Thus, in patients with primary STEMI, it may be relevant to evaluate function of both LV and RV.

Since LV inferior STEMI is a unique pathology with possible involvement of RV in MIs leading to RV dysfunction and worsen clinical outcomes, it would be reasonable to assess function of not only LV, but also RV in such patients.

The Study Objective

The purpose of the presented study is to evaluate prognostic importance of well-known EchoCG parameters (LV EF, LV MPI, RV MPI, TAPSE) and test the same for a sum of LV and RV MPIs against LV MPI or RV MPI alone and a combination of LV MPI and TAPSE against LV MPI or TAPSE alone in predicting early (hospital) and late (1-year) cardiac events in patients with patients with primary STEMI.

Materials and Methods

This study was approved by the local Ethics Committee of Yerevan State Medical University and all subjects were fully informed about the study and provided an informed consent to voluntary participate in the study.

Study Sample

296 patients with primary STEMI who underwent DMI at the Department of Urgent Cardiology of Erebouni Medical Centre, Yerevan in 1998-2011 were considered for study recruitment and 273 met eligibility criteria. The reasons for non-inclusion were the following diseases and conditions detected by history or typical symptoms that could bias the study findings - permanent or persistent atrial fibrillation; congenital heart diseases; significant rheumatic aortal and/or mitral stenoses; permanent pacemaker; strokes; diseases with severe PH; chronic kidney diseases; blood diseases and anemia and other metabolic and oncological diseases.

Of the 273 study patients, 240 (87.9%) were male and 33 (12.1%) were female. Age range was 38 to 72 years (mean 57.3±5.9 years) (table 3). A careful medical history for each of 273 enrolled patients was thoroughly assessed and a complete physical and standard instrumental and lab examination was performed on all the study subjects.

With regard to the diagnosis of STEMI and treatment strategy, patients were treated according to the institutional STEMI management algorithm based on the current evidence-based treatment guidelines [153-155]. 72 (26.4%) study subjects underwent primary PCI and the remaining 201 (83.6 %) received conservative treatment including 15 who received thrombolytic treatment.

Table 3. Baseline characteristics of the study population

Parameter	n	% ± SD
Males	240	87,9±5,4%
Age (mean ± SD years)		57,3±5,9
Co-diseases		
- Diabetes Milletus	71	26.0±7.2%
- Arterial Hypertension	103	37.7±8.0%
- Chronic Obstructive Pulmonary Diseases	91	33.3±7.8%
Reasrch Outcomes		
- In-hospital mortality	23	8.4±4.6%
- Early post-infarction angina	76	27.8±7.4%
- Ventricular Arrythmias	69	25.3±7.2%
- II-III° SA and/or AV blocks	65	23.8±7.0%
- Suprtaventricular Tachiarrythmias	25	9.2±4.8%
- Cargiogenic Shock	20	7.3±4.3%
- Pericardites	17	6.2±4.0%
- Successful reanimation cases	18	6.6±4.4%
- Post-hospital Death	21	9.1±4.4%
- Re-hospitalization	41	17.7±5.8%
RV involvement	131	48.0±8.3%
Primary PCI	72	26.4±7.3%

Note: To present frequencies of post-hospital death and re-hospitalization, calculations are based on the changed denominator of the sample size (cases of in-hospital death and missed data in one-year follow-up excluded)

Based on the data analysis method, we divided the study sample into different groups.

At first, to evaluate associations between means of EchoCG parameters and frequencies of clinical outcomes, the study sample was categorized into the following sets of groups:

- For the assessment of IHM: patients dead during the hospital period of time (n_+=23) vs. those discharged from the hospital (n_-=250);

- For the assessment of ACCs: a group with EPA ($n_+=76$) vs. a group without EPA ($n_-=197$), a group with VA ($n_+=69$) vs. a group without VA ($n_-=204$), a group with II-III^0 SA or AV blocks ($n_+=65$) vs. a group without HB ($n_-=208$), a group with SVT ($n_+=25$) vs. a group without SVT ($n_-=248$), a group with CS ($n_+=20$) vs. a group without CS ($n_-=253$), a group with PC ($n_+=17$) vs. a group without PC ($n_-=256$), and, finally, a group with SRC ($n_+=18$) vs. a group without SRC ($n_-=255$);
- For the assessment of PHD: patients dead during the post-infarction 1-year follow-up period of time ($n_+=21$) vs. the remaining patients ($n_-=211$);
- For the assessment of RH: patients re-hospitalized during the post-infarction 1-year follow-up period of time ($n_+=41$) vs. the remaining patients ($n_-=191$).

Second, based on LV MPI, RV MPI and TAPSE values, all 273 patients were categorized into the following groups:

- LV MPI ≥ 0.55 (n= 145) vs. LV MPI <0.55 (n=128);
- RV MPI ≥ 0.45 (n =120) vs. RV MPI <0.45 (n=153); and
- TAPSE ≤ 14 mm (n =142) vs. TAPSE >14 mm (n=131).

In addition to the above traditional EchoCG parameters, we tested any significant differences of frequencies of clinical outcomes between the following two subgroups:

- [LIMP+RIMP] ≥ 1.00 (n = 107) vs. [LIMP+RIMP] <1.00 (n=166).
- [LV MPI ≥ 0.55 and TAPSE ≤ 14 mm] (n = 105) vs. [LV MPI <0.55 and TAPSE >14 mm] (n = 168)

There were no statistically significant differences in the demographic characteristics and the preexisting morbidity among the study participants in the different study groups (assessed variables were age, AH, DM, and COPD).

Follow-up and Endpoints

For *the inpatient period, the following* research outcomes were thoroughly documented: cardiac death and any case of below listed ACCs: EPA, VA, II-III^0 SA and/or AV blocks, SVT, CS, PC and SRC. Patients were followed up for a median of 12 months for any occurrence of cardiac mortality and/or re-hospitalization due cardiac events.

Risk analysis of IHD and ACCs included all 273 patients of the study, yet the same of PHD and RH involved those 232 patients discharged from the hospital after primary STEMI and stayed under 1-year follow-up.

Calculation of EchoCG parameters by Pulsed Doppler Echocardiography

All DMI examinations and calculations of EchoCG parameters were performed with an ultrasound machine "Siemens G65" (Germany) within 24 hours of STEMI onset. DMI methodology was based on the American Society of Echocardiography's Guidelines [98, 156].

LV EF was measured according to Simpson's method as a ratio of the difference of LV end-diastolic and end-systolic volumes and the end-diastolic volume [157].

LV MPI was measured based on Doppler time intervals. It was calculated as the sum of the isovolumic contraction time and isovolumic relaxation time divided by the ejection time of LV (figure 8). The sum of isovolumic construction and relaxation times was determined by measuring the time from the end of atrial filling (end of A-wave) to the onset of atrial filling (onset of E-wave) minus ejection time. Ejection time was determined by measuring the LV-outflow velocity with the Pulsed Doppler in the 5-chamber apical view just below the aortic valve [158].

Figure 8. Schematic representation of the measurement of the LV Tei index (adopted by Lakoumentas J. et al, 2005)

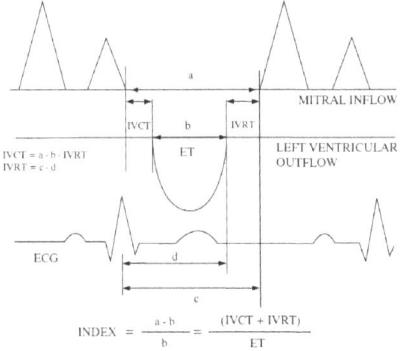

Note: a: time interval from the end to the start of transmitral flow, b: left ventricular ejection time (also denoted by ET), c: time interval from the peak of the R wave on the ECG to the start of transmitral flow, d: time interval from the peak of the R wave on the ECG to the end of ejection time, **ET:** (b) left ventricular ejection time, IVCT: isovolumic contraction time, IVRT: isovolumic relaxation time.

As for the **RV MPI**, ejection time was measured with pulsed Doppler of RV outflow (time from the onset to the cessation of flow), and the tricuspid (valve) closure-opening time was measured with the pulsed Doppler of the tricuspid inflow (time from the end of the transtricuspid A wave to the beginning of the transtricuspid E wave). RV MPI was calculated as the difference of tricuspid closure-opening and ejection times divided by ejection time (figure 9) [98].

Figure 9. Schematic representation of the measurement of the RV Tei index (adopted by Rudski L. et al, 2010)

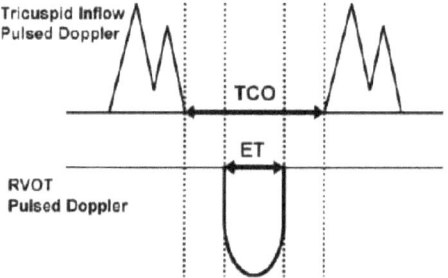

Explanation: The tricuspid (valve) closure opening time (TCO) encompasses isovolumic contraction time, ejection time (ET), and isovolumic relaxation time. In the pulsed Doppler method, TCO can also be measured by the duration of the tricuspid regurgitation continuous-wave Doppler signal. MPI = (TCO ET)/ET.

Within our study, we tested a new combined MPI of both ventricles as a simple sum of LV and RV MPIs.

To determine **TAPSE**, the apical four-chamber view was used, and an M-mode cursor was placed through the lateral tricuspid annulus in real time in such a way that the annulus moved along the M-mode cursor and the total displacement of the tricuspid annulus (in mm) from end-diastole to end-systole was measured (figure10) [39].

Figure 10. Schematic representation of the measurement of the TAPSE (adopted by Rudski L. et al, 2010)

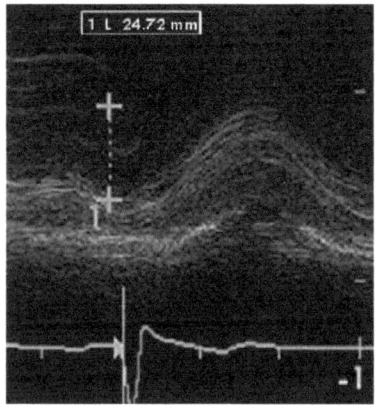

An experienced physician did both the DMI examinations and the reading of the images, unaware of the clinical data of the subjects.

Statistical Methods

Statistical analyses were performed with a statistical software program SPSS 17.0 (SPSS, Inc., Chicago, IL, USA).

Descriptive data summaries are presented with means and standard deviations (SD) or numbers (percentages). Bivariate analyses for the categorical outcome variables were conducted between groups using the χ^2 (chi-square) test.

Logistic regression was used to determine predictive values of each of EchoCG parameters. Covariate information (age, gender and clinical data regarding AH, DM, and COPD) was collected at the time of the EchoCG examination in all enrolled patients. Adjusted to all above covariates Odds Ratios (OR_{adj}) were calculated by applying binominal logistic regression model to evaluate the individual predictive importance of research parameters – LV MPI, RV MPI, a sum of LV and RV MPIs, and [LIMP + RIMP].

All statistical tests were two-sided, and tests with P-values of less than 0.05 were considered statistically significant. In the multivariate models, an independent variable was considered a significant predictor of the outcome variable (s) if the *p* value was less than 0.05.

Results

The study results are presented separately for LV EF, LV MPI, RV MPI, [LV MPI + RV MPI], TAPSE and [LIMP + RIMP].

A. Analysis of Means

LV Ejection Fraction: The mean of LV EF for the entire population was 45.3±2.1%. We found a statistically significant difference of LV EF only between CS(-) and (CS+) groups. This parameter was significantly lower in CS(+) than CS(-) group (42.2% vs 45.5%, p<0.05) (table 4).

Table 4. Comparative analysis of LV EF means between groups with and without clinical outcomes

Clinical outcomes	Event presence (+) LV EF mean%±SD%	Event absence (-) LV EF mean%±SD%	p value
IHD (n$_+$=23, n$_-$=250)	45.5±2.5%	45.2±2.4%	0.595
ACCs			
- EPA (n$_+$=76, n$_-$=197)	45.5 ±1.9%	45.2±2.2%	0.232
- VA (n$_+$=69, n$_-$=204)	44.7±2.5%	45.4±1.9%	0.091
- II-III^0 SA and/or AV HB (n$_+$=65, n$_-$=208)	45.0±2.1%	45.3±2.1%	0.353
- SVT (n$_+$=25, n$_-$=248)	45.3±1.9%	45.3±2.1%	0.953
- CS (n$_+$=20, n$_-$=253)	42.2±0.9%	45.5±2.0%	*p*<0.049
- PC (n$_+$=17, n$_-$=256)	45.1±1.8%	45.3±2.1%	0.778
- SRC (n$_+$=18, n$_-$=255)	46.0±1.6%	45.2±2.1%	0.118
PHD (n$_+$=21, n$_-$=211)	45.3±2.4%	45.2±2.1%	0.908
RH (n$_+$=41, n$_-$=191)	45.0±1.9%	45.3±2.1%	0.432

LV MPI: When comparing LV MPI means between groups of those with and without research outcomes in hospital period, we found statistically significant difference only for CS which was greater in patients who experienced this complication (p<0.001). Further, LV MPI was significantly greater in patients who died or re-hospitalized due cardiac events within 1st year of post-infarction follow-up ($p<0.001$ for both cases) (table 5).

Table 5. Comparative analysis of LV MPI means between groups with and without clinical outcomes

Clinical outcomes	Event presence (+) LV MPI mean±SD	Event absence (-) LV MPI mean±SD	p value
IHD (n_+=23, n_-=250)	0.57±0.07	0.56±0.07	0.379
ACCs			
- EPA (n_+=76, n_-=197)	0.56±0.07	0.56±0.07	0.467
- VA (n_+=69, n_-=204)	0.56±0.07	0.56±0.07	0.935
- II-III^0 SA and/or AV HB (n_+=65, n_-=208)	0.57±0.07	0.56±0.07	0.164
- SVT (n_+=25, n_-=248)	0.55±0.07	0.56±0.07	0.610
- CS (n_+=20, n_-=253)	0.64±0.08	0.56±0.06	$p<0.001$
- PC (n_+=17, n_-=256)	0.56±0.06	0.56±0.07	0.950
- SRC (n_+=18, n_-=255)	0.55±0.06	0.56±0.07	0.511
PHD (n_+=21, n_-=211)	0.65±0.07	0.55±0.07	$p<0.001$
RH (n_+=41, n_-=191)	0.61±0.10	0.55±0.06	$p<0.001$

RV MPI: The RV MPI of patients who died in hospital was significantly greater than that of those who were discharged from the hospital ($p<0.001$). As for ACCs during the inpatient stay, RV MPI was significantly greater in patients who experienced VA or CS ($p<0.001$ for both cases). Again, RV MPI was significantly greater in patients who dead or re-hospitalized in 1-year post-infarction follow-up ($p<0.007$ and $p<0.034$ respectively) (table 6).

Table 6. Comparative analysis of RV MPI means between groups with and without clinical outcomes

Clinical outcomes	Event presence (+) RV MPI mean±SD	Event absence (-) RV MPI mean±SD	p value
IHD (n_+=23, n_-=250)	0.49±0.07	0.42±0.08	$p<0.001$
ACCs			
- EPA (n_+=76, n_-=197)	0.41±0.08	0.43±0.08	0.082
- VA (n_+=69, n_-=204)	0.45±0.07	0.42±0.08	$p<0.001$
- II-III^0 SA and/or AV HB (n_+=65, n_-=208)	0.43±0.08	0.42±0.07	0.424
- SVT (n_+=25, n_-=248)	0.44±0.07	0.42±0.08	0.292
- CS (n_+=20, n_-=253)	0.51±0.05	0.42±0.07	$p<0.001$
- PC (n_+=17, n_-=256)	0.40±0.09	0.43±0.08	0.170
- SRC (n_+=18, n_-=255)	0.43±0.06	0.43±0.08	0.923
PHD (n_+=21, n_-=211)	0.47±0.05	0.42±0.08	$p<0.007$
RH (n_+=41, n_-=191)	0.45±0.06	0.42±0.08	$p<0.034$

TAPSE: The TAPSE of patients who died in hospital was significantly lower than that of those who were discharged from the hospital ($p<0.001$). As for in-hospital ACCs, TAPSE was significantly lower in patients who experienced VA, SVT or CS ($p<0.001$, $p<0.013$ and $p<0.001$ respectively). Contrary to the RV MPI , TAPSE mean does not statistically differ between patients who dead or re-hospitalized and who alive or do not re-hospitalized in 1-year post-infarction follow-up (table 7).

Table 7. Comparative analysis of TAPSE means between groups with and without clinical outcomes

Clinical outcomes	Event presence (+) TAPSE, mm mean±SD	Event absence (-) TAPSE, mm mean±SD	p value
IHD (n_+=23, n_-=250)	12.4±1.3	14.9±2.7	$p<0.001$
ACCs			
- EPA (n_+=76, n_-=197)	14.7±2.6	15.2±2.8	0.076
- VA (n_+=69, n_-=204)	13.0±2.0	15.2±2.6	$p<0.001$
- II-III^0 SA and/or AV HB (n_+=65, n_-=208)	14.6±2.6	14.8±2.8	0.464
- SVT (n_+=25, n_-=248)	14.5±2.6	15.8±2.6	$p<0.013$
- CS (n_+=20, n_-=253)	12.7±2.2	14.8±2.6	$p<0.001$
- PC (n_+=17, n_-=256)	14.6±2.7	15.5±2.9	0.055
- SRC (n_+=18, n_-=255)	14.6±2.7	15.5±2.5	0.077
PHD (n_+=21, n_-=211)	14.4±2.9	14.7±2.7	0.345
RH (n_+=41, n_-=191)	14.4±2.9	14.7±2.7	0.238

The sum of LV and RV MPI: The sum of LV and RV MPIs of patients who died in hospital was significantly greater than that of those who were discharged from the hospital ($p<0.003$). As for ACCs during the inpatient stay, the sum of LV and RV MPIs was significantly greater in patients who experienced VA or CS ($p<0.024$ and $p<0.001$ respectively). Similar to the RV MPI, the sum of LV and RV MPIs was significantly greater in patients who dead or re-hospitalized in 1-year post-infarction follow-up ($p<0.001$ for both cases) (table 8).

Table 8. Comparative analysis of [LV MPI + RV MPI] means between groups with and without clinical outcomes

Clinical outcomes	Event presence (+) LV MPI + RV MPI mean±SD	Event absence (-) LV MPI + RV MPI mean±SD	p value
IHD (n_+=23, n_-=250)	1.06±0.11	0.98±0.13	$p<0.003$
ACCs			
- EPA (n_+=76, n_-=197)	0.97±0.12	0.99±0.13	0.274
- VA (n_+=69, n_-=204)	1.02±0.12	0.98±0.13	$p<0.024$
- II-III^0 SA and/or AV HB (n_+=65, n_-=208)	1.00±0.14	0.98±0.12	0.213
- SVT (n_+=25, n_-=248)	1.00±0.12	0.99±0.13	0.721
- CS (n_+=20, n_-=253)	1.15±0.12	0.97±0.12	$p<0.001$
- PC (n_+=17, n_-=256)	0.96±0.13	0.99±0.13	0.388
- SRC (n_+=18, n_-=255)	0.98±0.11	0.99±0.13	0.762
PHD (n_+=21, n_-=211)	1.12±0.11	0.98±0.12	$p<0.001$
RH (n_+=41, n_-=191)	1.06±0.12	0.97±0.12	$p<0.001$

B. Risk analysis

In order to evaluate predictive importance of EchoCG parameters, we conducted both unadjusted and adjusted risk analysis between groups constructed by the cut-off values identified individually for each of those parameters (see Materials and Methods). We made such analysis for LV MPI, RV MPI, and TAPSE as well as newly introduced the sum of LV and RV MPIs and the combination of LV MPI and TAPSE.

LV MPI: Risk analysis between the group of patients with LV MPI$\geq$0.55 and LV MPI<0.55 revealed that LV MPI$\geq$0.55 can be seen as a prognostic factor to predict higher risks of CS in hospital treatment period and PHD and RH in one-year post-infarction follow-up (table 9). Particularly, LV MPI$\geq$0.55 increases probabilities of above three clinical outcomes by about 3.9 times ($p<0.022$), 5.0 times ($p<0.006$) and 2.8 times ($p<0.010$) correspondingly.

Table 9. Risk analysis between LV MPI≥0.55 and LV MPI<0.55 groups

Clinical outcomes	LV MPI≥0.55 %±SD (n_0=145, n_1=120)	LV MPI<0.55 %±SD (n_0=128, n_1=112)	p value of difference	OR_{adj}	95% confidence interval of OR_{adj}
IHD	10.3±3.7%	6.3±2.8%	0.224	-	-
ACCs					
- EPA	29.7±5.5%	25.8±4.9%	0.476	-	-
- VA	26.9±5.3%	23.4±4.8%	0.512	-	-
- II-III^0 SA and/or AV HB	24.8±5.2%	22.7±4.7%	0.674	-	-
- SVT	9.0±3.4%	9.4±3.3%	0.907	-	-
- CS	11.0±3.8%	3.1±2.0%	p<0.012	3.877	1.214-12.387
- PC	7.6±3.2%	4.7±2.4%	0.323	-	-
- SRC	6.9±3.1%	6.3±2.7%	0.830	-	-
PHD	13.3±3.7%	4.5±2.2%	p<0.019	5.005	1.583-15.826
RH	23.3±4.3%	11.6±3.4%	p<0.019	2.818	1.287-6.170

RV MPI: Risk analysis between the group of patients with RV MPI≥0.45 and EV MPI<0.45 revealed that RV MPI≥0.45 can be seen as a prognostic factor of predicting higher risks of IHD and CS in hospital treatment period (table 10). Particularly, RV MPI≥0.45 increases probabilities of above two clinical outcomes by about 2.6 times (p<0.022) and 4.5 times (p<0.006) correspondingly.

Table 10. Risk analysis between RV MPI≥0.45 and RV MPI<0.45 groups

Clinical outcomes	RV MPI≥0.45 %±SD (n_0=120, n_1=95)	RV MPI<0.45 %±SD (n_0=153, n_1=137)	p value of difference	OR_{adj}	95% confidence interval of OR_{adj}
IHD	12.5±3.6%	5.2±2.8%	p<0.032	2.530	1.842-5.904
ACCs					
- EPA	24.2±4.7%	30.7±5.7%	0.231	-	-
- VA	30.8±5.1%	20.9±5.0%	0.061	-	-
- II-III^0 SA and/or AV HB	28.3±4.9%	20.3±5.0%	0.120	-	-
- SVT	12.5±3.6%	6.5±3.1%	0.090	-	-
- CS	12.5±3.6%	3.3±2.2%	p<0.004	4.496	1.475-13.702
- PC	5.8±2.6%	6.5±3.1%	0.811	-	-
- SRC	8.3±3.0%	5.2±2.8%	0.305	-	-
PHD	11.6±3.1%	7.3±3.0%	0.264	-	-
RH	23.2±4.1%	13.9±4.0%	0.068	-	-

TAPSE: Risk analysis between the group of patients with TAPSE≤14 mm and TAPSE>14 mm revealed that TAPSE≤14 mm stands as a prognostic factor which predicts higher risks of IHD, VA and CS in hospital treatment period (table 11). Particularly, TAPSE≤14 increases probabilities of above three clinical outcomes by about 2.9 times (p<0.043), 2.7 times (p<0.001) and 3.6 times (p<0.020) correspondingly.

Table 11. Risk analysis between TAPSE≤14 mm and TAPSE>14 mm groups

Clinical outcomes	TAPSE≤14 mm %±SD (n_0=142, n_1=115)	TAPSE>14 mm %±SD (n_0=131, n_1=117)	p value of difference	OR_{adj}	95% confidence interval of OR_{adj}
IHD	12.0±3.9%	4.6±2.4%	$p<0.028$	2.875	1.034-7.998
ACCs					
- EPA	21.1±4.9%	27.5±5.1%	0.220	-	-
- VA	33.8±5.6%	16.0±4.2%	$p<0.001$	2.689	1.469 4.920
- II-III^0 SA and/or AV HB	26.1±5.2%	21.4±4.7%	0.364	-	-
- SVT	7.0±3.0%	11.5±3.6%	0.207	-	-
- CS	10.6±3.7%	3.8±2.2%	$p<0.033$	3.639	1.230-10.766
- PC	4.9±2.6%	7.6±3.0%	0.356	-	-
- SRC	6.3±4.9%	6.9±2.9%	0.859	-	-
PHD	11.3±3.4%	6.8±2.7%	0.236	-	-
RH	20.9±4.4%	14.5±3.8%	0.215	-	-

The sum of LV and RV MPIs: Risk analysis between the group of patients with the sum of LV and RV MPIs≥1.0 and <1.0 revealed that the sum of LV and RV MPIs≥1.0 can be seen as a prognostic factor which predicts higher risks of IHD, VA and CS in hospital treatment period as well as higher risks of PHD and RH in one-year post-infarction follow-up (table 12). Particularly, the sum of LV and RV MPIs≥1.0 increases the probability of IHD by about 2.2 times ($p<0.028$), VA – 4.5 times ($p<0.011$), CS – 4.8 times ($p<0.006$), PHD – 2.2 times ($p<0.012$) and RH – 3.0 times ($p<0.006$).

Table 12. Risk analysis between the sum of LV and RV MPIs≥1.0 and <1.0 groups

Clinical outcomes	The sum of LV and RV MPIs≥1.0 %±SD (n_0=107, n_1=83)	The sum of LV and RV MPIs<1.0 %±SD (n_0=166, n_1=149)	p value of difference	OR_{adj}	95% confidence interval of OR_{adj}
IHD	13.1±3.5%	5.4±2.9%	$p<0.026$	2.197	1.242-5.735
ACCs					
- EPA	26.2±4.5%	28.9±5.8%	0.621	-	-
- VA	32.7±4.9%	20.5±5.2%	$p<0.006$	1.619	1.096-2.926
- II-III^0 SA and/or AV HB	29.9±4.7%	19.9±5.1%	0.058	-	-
- SVT	12.1±3.4%	7.2±3.3%	0.169	-	-
- CS	14.0±3.6%	3.0±2.2%	$p<0.001$	4.793	1.582-14.518
- PC	6.5±2.6%	6.0±3.1%	0.863	-	-
- SRC	9.3±3.0%	4.8±2.8%	0.141	-	-
PHD	14.5±3.2%	6.0±2.9%	$p<0.032$	2.239	1.229-6.046
RH	27.7±4.1%	12.1±4.0%	$p<0.003$	3.031	1.369-6.709

The combination of LV MPI≥0.55 and TAPSE≤14 mm: Risk analysis between the group of patients with the combination of LV MPI≥0.55 and TAPSE≤14 mm and the remaining patients revealed that [LV MPI≥0.55 and TAPSE≤14 mm] criteria is a prognostic factor which predicts higher risks of IHD, VA and CS in hospital treatment period as well as higher risks of PHD and RH in one-year post-infarction follow-up (table 13). Particularly, [LV MPI≥0.55 and TAPSE≤14 mm] in a patient increases the probability of IHD by about 3.1 times ($p<0.021$), VA – 1.9 times ($p<0.024$), CS – 7.3 times ($p<0.001$), PHD – 3.5 times ($p<0.016$) and RH – 3.6 times ($p<0.001$).

Table 13. Risk analysis between the groups of patients with [LV MPI$\geq$0.55 and TAPSE$\leq$14mm] and remaining ones

Clinical outcomes	LV MPI$\geq$0.55 and TAPSE$\leq$14mm %$\pm$SD (n_0=105, n_1=80)	LV MPI<0.55 and/or TAPSE>14mm %$\pm$SD (n_0=168, n_1=152)	p value of difference	OR$_{adj}$	95% confidence interval of OR$_{adj}$
IHD	14.3$\pm$3.6%	4.8$\pm$2.8%	p<0.006	3.101	1.190-8.083
ACCs					
- EPA	28.6$\pm$6.6%	27.4$\pm$5.8%	0.831	-	-
- VA	32.4$\pm$4.8%	20.8$\pm$5.3%	p<0.033	1.859	1.135-2.946
- II-III^0 SA and/or AV HB	27.6$\pm$4.6%	21.4$\pm$5.3%	0.243	-	-
- SVT	12.4$\pm$3.4%	7.1$\pm$3.3%	0.144	-	-
- CS	14.3$\pm$3.6%	3.0$\pm$2.2%	p<0.001	7.283	2.402-22.084
- PC	6.7$\pm$2.6%	6.0$\pm$3.1%	0.797	-	-
- SRC	5.7$\pm$2.4%	7.1$\pm$3.3%	0.644	-	-
PHD	16.3$\pm$3.3%	5.3$\pm$2.8%	p<0.006	3.479	1.267-9.550
RH	30.0$\pm$4.1%	11.2$\pm$3.9%	p<0.001	3.637	1.678-7.884

Other findings: Bivariate logistic analysis allowed us evaluating other co-variables as well. For example, a patient age was a predictive factor for the CS (OR$_{adj}$=1.105, p<0.044) and PHD (OR$_{adj}$=1.177, p<0.003) when evaluating predictive importance of the sum of LV and RV MPIs$\geq$1.0.

C. Correlation analysis

Within this study, we also perform correlation analysis of EchoCG parameters to test their association either independence from well-known co-variables like age, gender, co-diseases as well as RV involvement (table 15). For that reason we used Spearman correlation coefficient (r_s) calculations to find out corresponding p values. We found no association between any of EchoCG criteria and considered co-variables, which allows us to state that all of above criteria are independent from age, gender, co-diseases as well as RVMI.

Table 14. Comparison of predictive values of different EchoCG parameters

Clinical outcomes	EchoCG Criteria				
	LV MPI ≥0.55	RV MPI ≥0.45	The sum of LV and RV MPIs ≥1.0	TAPSE ≤14 mm	[LV MPI≥0.55 and TAPSE≤14 mm]
	r_s	r_s	r_s	r_s	r_s
Age	(0.070)	(0.013)	(0.014)	0.110	(0.032)
Gender	0.011	(0.057)	(0.007)	0.086	0.030
DM	0.022	0.047	0.037	0.085	0.098
AH	(0.041)	(0.096)	(0.066)	(0.009)	0.006
COPD	0.019	0.072	0.052	(0.021)	0.064
RVMI	0.080	0.039	0.060	0.042	0.039

Discussion

It is accepted that LV EF is a good marker for predicting post-infarction complications, included HF. However, our data demonstrates that in patients with STEMI only CS is statistically associated with lower LV EF values and the remaining outcomes are not related with this EchoCG parameter. Published research studies have also proved that LV EF gets its prognostic importance especially for anterior rather than inferior wall MIs. Curtis et al. in a study showed that among HF patients in sinus rhythm, higher LV EFs are associated with a linear decrease in mortality [159]. Thus, for STEMIs, clinicians may need other prognostic criteria in estimating risks of cardiac death and other events. Our study suggests that other EchoCG parameters than LV EF (like LV and RV MPIs and TAPSE) are very likely to be useful for this purpose both right after the acute MIs and one-year post-infarction period.

Contrary to previous studies which evaluated predictive patterns of either the MPI (mostly – LV MPI) or TAPSE, we have investigated separately not only LV MPI, RV MPI and TAPSE, but also introduced and tested two more criteria which are a sum of LV and RV MPIs and a combination of LV MPI and TAPSE. Our study results allowed us concluding that each of above EchoCG parameters has its own prognostic importance for different – both early and late - periods of STEMIs.

We have demonstrated that LV MPI is a strong predictor of CS in hospital treatment period and of both PHD and RH in post-infarction one year of primary STEMIs. Our results proved that a criteria of LV MPI≥0.55 is strongly associated with about 3.9 times of increase in CS probability in hospital period of time ($p<0.022$) and about 5,0 times of increase in PHD and 2,8 times of increase in RH probabilities in one-year post-infarction period ($p<0.006$ and $p<0.010$ correspondingly).

Based on the published literature, the established prognostic usefulness of LV MPI remains somewhat controversial. While there are some studies underlining the role of LIMP in identifying patients with higher cardiac mortality or HF risk [117, 160-162], other researchers suggest that in the acute phase of MI, LV MPI measured at admission cannot reliably predict which patients are at high risk for in-hospital cardiac events [163-165].

To date, some research was done to define reference ranges of LV MPI for use in clinical practice. Ascione et al. established that LV MPI≥0.47 is useful in predicting which patients with first MI are at high risk for hospital cardiac events (death, HF, arrhythmias, or post-MI angina) [112]. Poulsen et al. showed that the LV MPI >0.45 in MI patients is the strongest independent predictor of the development of congestive HF [161]. Further, Møller et al. demonstrated that 1-year survival in first MI patients with LV MPI<0.63 was 89%, whereas in patients with LV MPI ≥0.63 it was 37% [117].

As with RV MPI, our study results demonstrated that this EchoCG parameter can stand for a strong predictor of CS in hospital treatment period and of both PHD and RH in post-infarction one year of primary STEMIs. Our results showed that a criteria of RV MPI≥0.45 is statistically related with about 2.5 times of increase in IHD risk and about 4.5 times of increase in CS risk in hospital period of time ($p<0.016$ and $p<0.008$ correspondingly).

As an estimator of the global RV function, RV MPI along with TAPSE and RV FAC was extensively researched for diseases and conditions accompanied with the PH. To date, however, a little is known on the usefulness of RV MPI in patients with

MI [107, 117]. For example, Vizzardi et al. demonstrated some association of RV MPI>0.38 and TAPSE< 18 mm values with 5 year total mortality and HF hospitalization in patients with chronic HG [166]. In another study, Chockalingam et al. [107] showed that in patients with STEMI RV MPI≥0.38 values have high sensitivity (82%) and specificity (95%) for the diagnosis of RVMI in the presence of acute MI and such a criterion can reliably diagnose RVMI.

Furthermore, our study not only outlines the usefulness of LV and/or RV MPIs as useful parameters for prediction of early or late cardiac events, but also introduces the combined sum of LV and RV MPIs as a "universal risk factor" for both early and late cardiac morbidity and mortality. We demonstrated that the sum of LV and RV MPIs≥1.0 is strongly associated with about 2.2 times of increase in IHD risk, 1.7 times of increase in VA risk about 4.8 times of increase in CS risk in hospital period of time ($p<0.028$, $p<0.011$, and $p<0.006$) as well as the same values increases both PHD and RH risks by about 2.2 and 3.0 times in one-year post-STEMI period ($p<0.012$ and $p<0.006$ correspondingly).

Thus, in our study, we demonstrated that Doppler measurements of both LV and RV functions are risk factors for cardiac events. MPIs provided prognostic information beyond that of currently established or existing measurements of cardiac function and conventional risk factors. Above all, we demonstrated that RV MPI determined within the first 24 hours of the STEMI onset enables noninvasive prediction of subsequent complications and early cardiac mortality. In addition, the study results indicated that predictive capacity of MPIs could be explained by the fact that LV MPI reflects global LV function, while RV MPI - global RV function, and the sum of LV and LV MPIs - combined global functions of both ventricles.

We explored the relevant literature and found no data that would compare predictive patterns of LV MPI and RV MPI, especially in patients with STEMI. Moreover, there was no published evidence that could examine the MPI indicator that combines both LIMP and RIMP.

The next traditional EchoCG parameter which we looking into was TAPSE. We found that this measurement is significantly associated with IHD and two ACCs (VA and CS). Our study results proved that the criteria of TAPSE≤14 mm is associated with about 2.9 times of increase in IHD risk, about 2,7 times of increase in VA risk and about 3,6 times of increase in CS in hospital treatment period of patients with primary STEMI ($p<0.043$, $p<0.001$ and $p<0.020$ correspondingly). Similar to the RV MPI, our findings via available literature were mainly related to non-ischemic diseases with PH syndrome. Only little data was available concerning some prognostic role of TAPSE in patients with MIs. Engström A. et al. showed that in STEMI patients presenting with CS on admission and treated with primary PCI, RV dysfunction as assessed by echocardiography (TAPSE≤14 mm) is an independent predictor for long-term mortality. In another study Antoni et el. demonstrated that RV function evaluated in terms of RV FAC (≥32%), TAPSE (<1.5 cm) and RV strain (≥−22.1%) provides strong prognostic information in patients treated with primary PCI for MIs [168].

Finally, we introduced a new prognostic criteria, a combination of LV MPI≥0.55 and TAPSE≤14 mm, which is very likely to be a strong predictor of both early and late cardiac events. For in-hospital treatment period of STEMIs, above parameter is associated with about 3.1 times of increase in IHD risk, 1,9 times of increase in VA risk and 7.3 times of increase in CS risk ($p<0.021$, $p<0.024$ and $p<0.001$ correspondingly). Again, for one-year post-infarction follow-up, the same combined parameter predicts about 3.5 times of increase in PHD and 3.6 times of increase in RH risks ($p<0.016$ and $p<0.001$ correspondingly). Thus this new criteria is very likely to combine early and late prognostic patterns of TAPSE and LV MPI.

When looking into comparative prognostic influences of above mentioned EchoCG parameters, it becomes clear that for some clinical outcomes the combined [LV MPI≥0.55 and TAPSE≤14 mm] has explicit advantages as it has greater "influence size" and/or higher significance (table 14). For example, the suggested [LV MPI≥0.55 and TAPSE≤14 mm] is the best criteria to predict IHD, CS in the hospital treatment period and RH in one-year post-infarction follow-up period while the sum of LV MPIs≥0.55 seems to be preferable to predict one-year PHD, and TAPSE≤14 mm – for VA.

Table 14. Comparison of predictive values of different EchoCG criteria

Clinical outcomes	EchoCG Criteria				
	LV MPI $\geq$0,55	RV MPI $\geq$0,45	The sum of LV and RV MPIs $\geq$1,0	TAPSE $\leq$14 mm	[LV MPI$\geq$0.55 and TAPSE$\leq$14 mm]
	OR$_{adj}$ (p)	OR$_{adj}$ (p)	OR$_{adj}$ (p)	OR$_{adj}$ (p)	OR$_{adj}$ (p)
IHD	-	2.530 (p<0.016)	2.197 (p<0.028)	2.875 (p<0.043)	3.101 (p<0.021)
ACCs					
- EPA	-	-	-	-	-
- VA	-	-	1.691 (p<0.011)	2.689 (p<0.001)	1.859 (p<0.024)
- II-III^0 SA and/or AV HB	-	-	-	-	-
- SVT	-	-	-	-	-
- CS	3.877 (p<0.022)	4.496 (p<0.008)	4.793 (p<0.006)	3.639 (p<0.020)	7.283 (p<0.001)
- PC	-	-	-	-	-
- SRC	-	-	-	-	-
PHD	5.005 (p<0.006)	-	2.239 (p<0.012)	-	3.479 (p<0.016)
RH	2.818 (p<0.010)	-	3.031 (p<0.006)	-	3.637 (p<0.001)

Study Limitations

The main limitation of the present study relates to the relatively small sample size of the patient population. This study also lacked measurements of other EchoCG parameters of LV and RV function, which also may be useful predictors of adverse outcomes in STEMI patients. Therefore, with the above-mentioned limitations, long-term follow-up and large-scale prospective studies are needed to further confirm the predictive value of the suggested combined parameter and support our findings.

Conclusions

The sum of LV and RV MPIs as well as a combination of LV MPI and TAPSE appear to be clinically relevant measurements of both ventricles' global function and may prove to be valuable tools in assessing the risk of both early and late cardiac morbidity and mortality. Thus, as useful add-ons to well-known traditional EchoCG parameters, we suggest using the the the sum of MPIs of both ventricles of ≥ 1.0 as well as a combination of LV MPI≥ 0.55 and TAPSE≤ 14 mm for identifying high risk patients in hospital and 1-year post-infarction periods in patients with primary STEMI. Combination of LV MPI and TAPSE measured right after primary STEMI appeared to be superior to the same parameters alone for the early risk stratification of patients for early and late cardiac events and could facilitate in the identification of patients who are at risk for adverse cardiac events both in hospital treatment regimen and one year after MI. Quantitative assessment of LV and RV functions with LV MPIs and TAPSE may improve the risk stratification of patients after primary STEMIs. Thus, our study highlights the necessity to focus more attention on early routine assessment of RV along with LV myocardial function in the follow-up of primary STEMI patients.

References

1. Harvey W. Exercitatio Anatomica de Motu Cordis et Sanguinis in Animalibus. 1628.
2. Goldstein J. The right ventricle: what's right and what's wrong. Coron Artery Dis. 2005; 16:1-3.
3. Zaffran S., Kelly R., Meilhac S., Buckingham M., Brown N. Right ventricular myocardium derives from the anterior heart field. Circ Res. 2004; 95:261-268.
4. Rigolin V., Robiolio P., Wilson J., Harrison J., Bashore T. The forgotten chamber: the importance of the right ventricle. Cathet Cardiovasc Diagn. 1995 May;35(1):18-28.
5. Badano L. The EAE Textbook of Echocardiography. European Society of Cardiology ed. E. by. 2011: Oxford University Press.
6. Tourneau T., Piriou N., Donal E., Deswarte G., Topilsky Y., et al. Imaging and modern assessment of the right ventricle. Minerva Cardioangiol, 2011 Aug;59(4): p. 349-73
7. Bleasdale R., Frenneaux M. Prognostic importance of right ventricular dysfunction Heart 2002;88:323-324.
8. Noordegraa, A., Galiè N. The role of the right ventricle in pulmonary arterial hypertension. Eur Respir Rev, 2011 20(122): 243-253.
9. Sallach, J., Tang W., Borowski A., Tong W., Porter T. et al. Right atrial volume index in chronic systolic heart failure and prognosis. JACC Cardiovasc Imaging, 2009. 2:527-34.
10. Vecchia L., Zanolla L., Varotto L. Reduced right ventricular ejection fraction as a marker for idiopathic dilated cardiomyopathy compared with ischemic left ventricular dysfunction. Am Heart J, 2001. 142:181-9.
11. Moazami N., Hill L., Right ventricular dysfunction in patients with acute inferior MI: role of RV mechanical support. Thorac Cardiovasc Surg, 2003 Oct;51(5):290-2.
12. Dell'Italia L. Anatomy and Physiology of the Right Ventricle. Cardiology Clinics, 2012. 30(2):167-87.
13. Sanders A. Coronary thrombosis with complete heart-block and relative ventricular tachycardia a case report. Am Heart J, 1931(6):820-3.
14. Cohn J., Guiha N., Broder M., Limas C. Right ventricular infarction: Clinical and hemodynamic features. Am J Cardiol, 1974. 33: p. 209-214.

15. Hsu S., Lin J., Chang S. Right ventricular function in patients with different infarction sites after a first acute myocardial infarction. Am J Med Sci, 2011 Dec;342(6): 474-9.

16. Voelkel N., Quaife R., Leinwand L., Barst R., McGoon R., et al. Right Ventricular Function and Failure: Report of a National Heart, Lung, and Blood Institute Working Group on Cellular and Molecular Mechanisms of Right Heart Failure. Circulation, 2006; 114:1883-1891.

17. Pinsky M. Assessment of indices of preload and volume responsiveness. Curr Opin Crit Care, 2005(11):235-239.

18. Foale R., Nihoyannopoulos P., McKenna W., Kleinebenne A., Nadazdin A., et al. Echocardiographic measurement of the normal adult right ventricle. Br Heart J 1986;56:33-44.

19. Ho S., Nihoyannopoulos P. Anatomy, echocardiography, and normal right ventricular dimensions. Heart. Apr 2006; 92(Suppl 1): i2-i13.

20. Goor D., Lillehei C. Congenital malformations of the heart, 1st edn. Grune and Stratton, 1975 New York, p. 1-37.

21. Lindqvist P., Calcuttea A., Henein M. Echocardiography in the assessment of right heart function 2008. Eur J Echocardiogr 9:225–234.

22. Haddad F., Hunt S., Rosenthal D., Murphy D. Right ventricular function in cardiovascular disease, part I: anatomy, physiology, aging, and functional assessment of the right ventricle. Circulation, 2008. 117:1436-48.

23. Dell'Italia LJ. The right ventricle: anatomy, physiology, and clinical importance. Curr Probl Cardiol. 1991; 16: 653–720.

24. Kukulski T., Hubbert L., Arnold M., Wranne B., Hatle L., et al. Normal regional right ventricular function and its change with age: a Doppler myocardial imaging study. J Am Soc Echocardiogr. 2000; 13: 194–204

25. Davidson C., Bonow R. Cardiac catheterization. In: Zipes D, Libby P, Bonow R, Braunwald E, eds. Braunwald's Heart Disease: A Textbook of Cardiovascular Medicine. 7th ed. Philadelphia, Pa: Elsevier; 2005: chap ll.

26. Lumens J., Arts T., Marcus J., Vonk-Noordegraaf A., et al., Early-Diastolic Left Ventricular Lengthening Implies Pulmonary Hypertension-Induced Right Ventricular Decompensation. Cardiovasc Res. 2012 Nov 1;96(2):286-95.

27. Osculati G., Malfatto G., Chianca R., Perego GB. Left-to-right systolic ventricular interaction in patients undergoing biventricular stimulation for dilated cardiomyopathy. J Appl Physiol, 2010(109):418-423.

28. Jerzewski A., Steendijk P., Pattynama PM., Leeuwenburgh BP., de Roos A., et al. Right ventricular systolic function and ventricular interaction during acute embolisation of the left anterior descending coronary artery in sheep. Cardiovasc Res 43: 86–95, 1999.

29. Li K., Santamore W. Contribution of each wall to biventricular function. Cardiovasc Res 27: 792–800, 1993.

30. Maughan WL., Sunagawa K., Sagawa K. Ventricular systolic interdependence: volume elastance model in isolated canine hearts. Am J Physiol Heart Circ Physiol 253: H1381–H1390, 1987.

31. Yamaguchi S., Harasawa H., Li KS., Zhu D., Santamore WP. Comparative significance in systolic ventricular interaction. Cardiovasc Res, 1991. 25:774-83.

32. Simon M., Pinsky M. Right ventricular dysfunction and failure in chronic pressure overload. Cardiol Res Pract, 2011 Mar 23: 2011.

33. Dell'Italia L., Walsh R. Application of a time varying elastance model to right ventricular performance in man. Cardiovasc Res. 1988; 22: 864–874.

34. Suga H., Sagawa K., Shoukas A. Load independence of the instantaneous pressure-volume ratio of the canine left ventricle and effects of epinephrine and heart rate on the ratio. Circ Res. 1973; 32: 314–322.

35. Starling M., Walsh R., Dell'Italia L., Mancini G., Lasher J., et al. The relationship of various measures of end-systole to left ventricular maximum time-varying elastance in man. Circulation. 1987; 76: 32–43.

36. Naeije R. Pulmonary vascular function. In: Peacock AJ, Rubin LJ, ed. Pulmonary Circulation. London: Arnold; 2004. p 3-11.

37. Chin K., Kim N., Rubin L. The right ventricle in pulmonary hypertension.Coron Artery Dis. 2005; 16:13–18.

38. Yu C., Sanderson J., Chan S., Yeung L., Hung Y., et al. Right ventricular diastolic dysfunction in heart failure. Circulation. 1996; 93:1509-1514.

39. Burgess M., Mogulkoc N., Bright-Thomas R., Bishop P., Egan J., et al. Comparison of echocardiographic markers of right ventricular function in determining prognosis in chronic pulmonary disease. J Am Soc Echocardiogr.2002; 15:633-639.

40. Gaasch W., Cole J., Quinones M., Alexander J. Dynamic determinants of left ventricular diastolic pressure-volume relations in man. Circulation. 1975;51: 317–323.

41. Smithuis R., Willems T. Coronary anatomy and anomalies. The Radiology Assistant, 2008(23): 12-1.

42. Brown G. Vascular pattern of myocardium of right ventricle of human heart. Br Heart J. 1968; 30: 679–686.

43. Kinch J., Ryan T. Right ventricular infarction. N Engl J Med. 1994; 330:1211-1217.

44. Farb A, Burke AP, Virmani R. Anatomy and pathology of the right ventricle (including acquired tricuspid and pulmonic valve disease). Cardiol Clin. 1992;10:1-21.

45. Haupt H., Hutchins G., Moore G. Right ventricular infarction: role of the moderator band artery in determining infarct size. Circulation. 1983; 67:1268–1272.

46. Fuster V., Alexander R., O'Rourke R. Hurst's The Heart (10th ed.). McGraw-Hill 2001. p. 53.

47. Janik M., Chappell C., Green T., Kacharava A. Two coincident coronary anomalies: absent left main coronary artery and origin of the right coronary artery from the middle left anterior descending artery. Tex Heart Inst J. 2009;36(2):180-1.

48. Garty I., Barzilay J., Bloch L., Antonelli D., Koltun B. The diagnosis and early complications of right ventricular infarction. Eur J Nucl Med. 1984;9(10):453-60.

49. McDaniel M., Willis P., Walker B. Plaque necrotic core content is greater immediately distal to bifurcations compared to bifurcations in the proximal lad of patients with CAD. Am J Cardiol, 2008. 102(8).

50. Giannitsis E., Potratz J., Wiegand U., Stierle U., Djonlagic H., et al. Impact of early accelerated dose tissue plasminogen activator on in-hospital patency of the infarcted vessel in patients with acute right ventricular infarction. Heart. Jun 1997;77(6):512-6.

51. Herrera E. Acute infarction of the right ventricle. Physiopathology, treatment, and prognosis [Article in Spanish]. Arch Cardiol Mex, 2001 Jan-Mar;71(Suppl 1): S111-3.

52. Haupt H., Hutchins G., Moore G. Right ventricular infarction: role of the moderator band artery in determining infarct size. Circulation. Jun 1983;67(6):1268-72.

53. Hurst J. Comments about the electrocardiographic signs of right ventricular infarction. Clin Cardiol. Apr 1998;21(4):289-91.

54. Andersen H., Falk E., Nielsen D. Right ventricular infarction: frequency, size and topography in coronary heart disease: a prospective study comprising 107

consecutive autopsies from a coronary care unit. J AM COLL CARDIOL. Dec 1987;10(6):1223-32.

55. Goldstein J., Barzilai B., Rosamond T., Eisenberg P., Jaffe A. Determinants of hemodynamic compromise with severe right ventricular infarction. Circulation1990;82:359–368.

56. Kinn J., Ajluni S., Samyn J., Bates E., Grines C., et al. Rapid hemodynamic improvement after reperfusion during right ventricular infarction. J AM COLL CARDIOL. Nov 1 1995;26(5):1230-4.

57. Bates E. Revisiting reperfusion therapy in inferior myocardial infarction. J AM COLL CARDIOL. Aug 1997;30(2):334-42.

58. Wartman WB, Hellerstein HK: The incidence of heart disease in 2,000 consecutive autopsies. Ann Intern Med1948;28:41-65.

59. Isner J., Roberts W. Right ventricular infarction secondary to coronary heart disease: Frequency, locations, associated findings and significance from analysis of 236 necropsy patients with acute or healed myocardial infarction. Am J Cardiol1978;42:885-894.

60. Lopez-Sendon J., Coma-Canella I., Gamallo C. Sensitivity and specificity of hemodynamic criteria in the diagnosis of acute right ventricular infarction. Circulation1981;64:515–525.

61. Shah P., Maddahi J., Berman D., Pichler M., Swan H. Scintigraphically detected predominant right ventricular dysfunction in acute myocardial infarction: Clinical and hemodynamic correlates and implications for therapy and prognosis. J Am Coll Cardiol 1985;6:1264-1272.

62. Andersen H., Nielsen D., Falk E. Right ventricular infarction: larger enzyme release with posterior than with anterior involvement. Int J Cardiol. Mar 1989;22(3):347-55.

63. Andersen H., Nielsen D., Lund O., Falk E. Prognostic significance of right ventricular infarction diagnosed by ST elevation in right chest leads V3R to V7R. INT J CARDIOL. Jun 1989;23(3):349-56.

64. Birnbaum Y., Wagner G., Barbash G., Gates K., Criger D., et al. Correlation of angiographic findings and right (V1 to V3) versus left (V4 to V6) precordial ST-segment depression in inferior wall acute myocardial infarction. AM J CARDIOL. Jan 15 1999;83(2):143-8.

65. Bowers T., O'Neill W., Goldstein J., Grines C., Pica M., et al. Effect of reperfusion on biventricular function and survival after right ventricular infarction. N Engl J Med1998;338:933-940.

66. Braat S., Brugada P., den Dulk K., van Ommen V., Wellens HJ Value of lead V4R for recognition of the infarct coronary artery in acute inferior myocardial infarction. Am J Cardiol. Jun 1 1984;53(11):1538-41.

67. Goldstein J., Vlahakes G., Verrier E., Schiller N., Botvinick E., et al. Volume loading improves low cardiac output in experimental right ventricular infarction. J Am Coll Cardiol1983;2:270-278.

68. Siniorakis E., Nikolaou N., Sarantopoulos C., Sotirelos K., Iliopoulos N., et al. Volume loading in predominant righ ventricular infarction: Bedside hemodynamics using rapid response thermistors. Eur Heart J1994;15:1340-1347.

69. Brookes C., Ravn H., White P., Moeldrup U., Oldershaw P., et al. Acute right ventricular dilatation in response to ischemia significantly impairs left ventricular systolic performance. Circulation 1999;100:761-767.

70. Cintron G., Hernandez E., Linares E., Aranda J. Bedside recognition, incidence and clinical course of right ventricular infarction. Am J Cardiol1981;47:224-227.

71. Shiraki H, Niaki M., MD,1 Marzbali N., Salehiomran M., Acute impact of right ventricular infarction on early hemodynamic course after inferior myocardial infarction. Circulation, 2010 74(1): 148-55.

72. Jacobs A., Leopold J., Bates E., Mendes L., Sleeper L., et al. Cardiogenic shock caused by right ventricular infarction: A report from the SHOCK registry. Journal of the American College of Cardiology 2003; 41(8):1273-1279.

73. Goldstein J., Vlahakes G., Verrier E. The role of right ventricular systolic dysfunction and elevated intrapericardial pressure in the genesis of low output in experimental right ventricular infarction. Circulation 1982; 65:513–522.

74. Ratliff N., Hackel D. Combined right and left ventricular infarction: pathogenesis and clinicopathologic correlations. Am J Cardiol 1980; 45:217-221.

75. Lee F. Hemodynamics of the right ventricle in normal and diseased states, Cardiol Clin 1992;10:59-67.

76. Dell'Italia LJ, Starling MR, O'Rourke RA: Physical examination for exclusion of hemodynamically important right ventricular infarction. Ann Intern Med 1983;99:608-611.

77. Takeuchi M., Minamiji K., Fujino M., Kurogane H., Yamada S., et al. Role of right ventricular asynergy and tricuspid regurgitation in hemodynamic

alterations during acute inferior myocardial infarction. Jpn Heart J 1989;305:615–625.

78. Braat S., deZwaan C., Brugada P., Coenegracht J., Wellens H. Right ventricular involvement with acute inferior wall myocardial infarction identifies high risk of developing atrioventricular nodal conduction disturbances. Am Heart J 1984;107:1183–1187.

79. Malla R., Sayami A. In hospital complications and mortality of patients of inferior wall myocardial infarction with right ventricular infarction. JNMA J Nepal Med Assoc, 2007 Jul-Sep;46(167):99-102.

80. Hayrapetyan H., Adamyan K., Arakelyan I. Life-threatening cardiac complications in patients with acute inferior STEMI with right ventricular involvement. European Heart Journal: Acute Cardiovascular Care Abstract Supplement 2013; 1(S2):29.

81. Moye S., Carney M., Holstege C., Mattu A., Brady W. The electrocardiogram in right ventricular myocardial infarction. Am J Emerg Med. 2005;23:793-9.

82. Somers M., Brady W., Bateman D., Mattu A., Perron A. Additional electrocardiographic leads in the ED chest pain patient: Right ventricular and posterior leads. Am J Emerg Med. 2003;21:563-73.

83. Robalino B., Whitlow P., Underwood D., Salcedo E. Electrocardiographic manifestations of right ventricular infarction. Am Heart J. 1989;118:138-44.

84. Zehender M., Kasper W., Kauder E. Right ventricular infarction as an independent predictor of prognosis after acute inferior myocardial infarction. N Engl J Med. 1993;328:981-8.

85. Yoshino H., Udagawa H., Shimizu H. ST-segment elevation in right precordial leads implies depressed right ventricular function after acute inferior myocardial infarction. Am Heart J. 1998;135:689-95.

86. Ondrus T., Kanovsky J., Novotny T., Andrsova I., Spinar J., et al. Clinical Cardiology: Review Right ventricular myocardial infarction: From pathophysiology to prognosis. Exp Clin Cardiol. 2013 Winter; 18(1): 27-30.

87. O'Rourke R., Dell'Italia L. Diagnosis and management of right ventricular myocardial infarction. Curr Probl Cardiol. 2004;29:6-47.

88. Zaborska B., Makowska E., Pilichowska E., Maciejewski P., Bednarz B., et al. The diagnostic and prognostic value of right ventricular myocardial velocities in inferior myocardial infarction treated with primary percutaneous intervention. Kardiol Pol, 2011. 69(10):1054-61.

89. Lopez-Sendon J., Garcia-Fernandez M., Coma-Canella I., Yanguela M., Banuelos F. Segmental right ventricular function after acute myocardial infarction: Two-dimensional echocardiographic study in 63 patients. J Am Coll Cardiol 1983;51:390–396.

90. Hoffmann R., Hanrath P. Tricuspid annular velocity measurement. Simple and accurate solution for a delicate problem? Eur Heart J 2001;22:280-2.

91. Henein M., O'Sullivan C., Coats A., Gibson D. Angiotens in converting enzyme (ACE) inhibitors revert abnormal right ventricular filling in patients with restrictive left ventricular disease. J Am Coll Cardiol 1998;32:1187-93.

92. Lindqvist P., Henein M., Kazzam E. Right ventricular outflow tract fractional shortening: an applicable measure of right ventricular systolic function. Eur J Echocardiogr 2003;4:29-35.

93. Lindqvist P., Olofsson B., Backman C., Suhr O., Waldenstrom A. Pulsed tissue Doppler and strain imaging discloses early signs of infiltrative cardiac disease: a study on patients with familial amyloidotic polyneuropathy. Eur J Echocardiogr 2006;7:22-30.

94. Vignon P., Weinert L., Mor-Avi V., Spencer K., Bednarz J., et al. Quantitative assessment of regional right ventricular function with color kinesis. Am J Respir Crit Care Med 1999;159:1949-59.

95. Casazza F., Bongarzoni A., Capozi A., Agostoni O. Regional right ventricular dysfunction in acute pulmonary embolism and right ventricular infarction. Eur J Echocardiogr 2005;6:11-4.

96. Greil G., Beerbaum P., Razavi R., Miller O. Imaging the right ventricle: non-invasive imaging. Heart, 2008; 94:803-8.

97. Kircher B., Himelman R., Schiller N. Noninvasive estimation of right atrial pressure from the inspiratory collapse of the inferior vena cava. Am J Cardiol 1990;66:493-6

98. Rudski L., Lai W., Afilalo J., Hua L., Handschumacher M., et al. Guidelines for the Echocardiographic Assessment of the Right Heart in Adults: A Report from the American Society of Echocardiography, Endorsed by the European Association of Echocardiography, a registered branch of the European Society of Cardiology, and the Canadian Society of Echocardiography. J Am Soc Echocardiogr, 2010. 23:685-713

99. Cohen A., Logeart D., Chauvel C. Right ventricular infarction. N Engl J Med. 1998;339:479-80.

100. Zornoff L., Skali H., Pfeffer M., St John S., Rouleau J., et al. Right ventricular dysfunction and risk of heart failure and mortality after myocardial infarction. J Am Coll Cardiol 2002;39:1450-5.

101. Anavekar N., Skali H., Bourgoun M., Ghali J., Kober L., et al. Usefulness of right ventricular fractional area change to predict death, heart failure, and stroke following myocardial infarction (from the VALIANT ECHO study). Am J Cardiol 2008;101:607-12.

102. Kaul S., Tei C., Hopkins J., Shah P. Assessment of right ventricular function using two-dimensional echocardiography. Am Heart J 1984;107: 526-31.

103. Tamborini G., Pepi M., Galli C., Maltagliati A., Celeste F., et al. Feasibility and accuracy of a routine echocardiographic assessment of right ventricular function. Int J Cardiol 2007;115:86-9.

104. Tei C., Nishimura R., Seward J., Tajik A. Noninvasive Doppler-derived myocardial performance index: correlation with simultaneous measurements of cardiac catheterization measurements. Echocardiogr, 1997(10): p. 169-178

105. Tei C., Dujardin K., Hodge D., Bailey K., McGoon M., et al. Doppler echocardiographic index for assessment of global right ventricular function. J Am Soc Echocardiogr 1996;9:838-47.

106. Yoshifuku S., Otsuji Y., Takasaki K., Yuge K., Kisanuki A., et al. Pseudonormalized Doppler total ejection isovolume (Tei) index in patients with right ventricular acute myocardial infarction. Am J Cardiol 2003;91:527-31.

107. Chockalingam A., Gnanavelu G., Alagesan R., Subramaniam T. Myocardial performance index in evaluation of acute right ventricular myocardial infarction. Echocardiography 2004;21:487-94.

108. Sebbag I., Rudski L., Therrien J., Hirsch A., Langleben D. Effect of chronic infusion of epoprostenol on echocardiographic right ventricular myocardial performance index and its relation to clinical outcome in patients with primary pulmonary hypertension. Am J Cardiol 2001; 88:1060-3.

109. Abd El Rahman M., Abdul-Khaliq H., Vogel M., Alexi-Meskischvili V., Gutberlet M., et al. Value of the new Doppler-derived myocardial performance index for the evaluation of right and left ventricular function following repair of tetralogy of Fallot. Pediatr Cardiol 2002; 23:502-7.

110. Schwerzmann M., Samman A., Salehian O., Holm J., Provost Y., et al. Comparison of echocardiographic and cardiac magnetic resonance imaging for assessing right ventricular function in adults with repaired tetralogy of Fallot. Am J Cardiol 2007;99:1593-7.

111. Biering-Sørensen T., Mogelvang R., Søgaard P., Pedersen S., Galatius S., et al., Prognostic Value of Cardiac Time Intervals by Tissue Doppler Imaging M-Mode in Patients with Acute ST Segment Elevation Myocardial Infarction Treated with Primary Percutaneous Coronary Intervention. Circ Cardiovasc Imaging, 2013; 6:457-465.

112. Ascione L., Michele M., Accadia M., Rumolo S., Damiano L., et al. Myocardial global performance index as a predictor of in-hospital cardiac events in patients with first myocardial infarction. J Am Soc Echocardiogr, 2003 Oct;16(10):1019-23.

113. Kuwahara E., Otsuji Y., and Takasaki K. Increased Tei index suggests absence of adequate coronary reperfusion in patients with first anteroseptal acute myocardial infarction. Circulation, 2006. 70:248-253.

114. Rahman N., Kazmi K., and Yousaf M. Non-invasive prediction of ST elevation myocardial infarction complications by left ventricular Tei index. J Pak Med Assoc, 2009 Feb;59(2):75-8.

115. Celić V., Dekleva M., Majstorović A., Radivojević N., Kostić N., et al., Myocardial performance index: prediction and monitoring of remodeling and functioning of the left ventricle after first myocardial infarction [Article in Serbian]. Med Pregl, 2010 Sep-Oct;63(9-10):652-5.

116. Carluccio E., Biagioli P., Alunni G., Murrone A., Zuchi C., et al., Improvement of myocardial performance (Tei) index closely reflects intrinsic improvement of cardiac function: assessment in revascularized hibernating myocardium. Echocardiography, 2012 Mar;29(3):298-306.

117. Møller J., Pellikka P., Hillis G., Oh J.Prognostic importance of systolic and diastolic function after acute myocardial infarction. Am Heart J, 2003(145):147-153.

118. Szymanski P., Rezler J., Stec S., Budaj A. Long-term prognostic value of an index of myocardial performance in patients with myocardial infarction. Clin Cardiol, 2002(25):378-383

119. Jensen C., Jochims M., Hunold P., Sabin G., Schlosser T., et al. Right ventricular involvement in acute left ventricular myocardial infarction: prognostic implications of MRI findings. Am J Roentgenol 2010; 194: 592–598.

120. Kumar A., Abdel-Aty H., Kriedemann I., Schulz-Menger J., Gross C., et al. Contrast-enhanced cardiovascular magnetic resonance imaging of right ventricular infarction. J Am Coll Cardiol 2006; 48: 1969–1976

121. Inohara T. The challenges in the management of right ventricular infarction European Heart Journal: Acute Cardiovascular Care 2048872613490122, first published on May 21, 2013.

122. Goldstein J. Right heart ischemia: pathophysiology, natural history, and clinical management. Prog Cardiovasc Dis 1998; 40: 325–341.

123. Horan L. and Flowers N. Right ventricular infarction: specific requirements of management. Am Fam Physician 1999; 60: 1727–1734.

124. Owens C., McClelland A., Walsh S. In-hospital percutaneous coronary intervention improves in-hospital survival in patients with acute inferior myocardial infarction particularly with right ventricular involvement. J Invasive Cardiol 2009; 21: 40–44.

125. Dell'Italia L., Starling M., Blumhardt R., Lasher J., O'Rourke R. Comparative effects of volume loading, dobutamine, and nitroprusside in patients with predominant right ventricular infarction. Circulation 1985; 72: 1327–1335.

126. Ferrario M., Poli A., Previtali M., Lanzarini L., Fetiveau R., et al. Hemodynamics of volume loading compared with dobutamine in severe right ventricular infarction. Am J Cardiol 1994; 74: 329–333.

127. Berisha S., Kastrati A., Goda A., Popa Y. Optimal value of filling pressure in the right side of the heart in acute right ventricular infarction. BMJ 1990; 63: 98–1.

128. Goldstein J. Pathophysiology and management of right heart ischemia. J Am Coll Cardiol.2002;40:841–5.

129. Adamyan K., Hayrapetyan H. Clinical effectiveness of primary PCI and its influence on prognosis in left ventricle inferior wall ST elevated myocardial infarction with involvement of right ventricle [in Russian]. Preventive Medicine 2013 2:39-44.

130. Hayrapetyan H. Primary PCI in patients with left ventricle inferior wall ST elevated myocardial infarction with or without involvement of right ventricle [in Russian]. International scientific-research journal 2013; 7(14),5:10-14.

131. Assali A., Teplitsky I., Ben-Dor I., Solodky A., Brosh D., et al. Prognostic importance of right ventricular infarction in an acute myocardial infarction cohort referred for contemporary percutaneous reperfusion therapy. Am Heart J 2007; 153: 231–237.

132. Kapur N., Paruchuri V., Korabathina R., Al-Mohammdi R., Mudd J., et al. Effects of a percutaneous mechanical circulatory support device for medically refractory right ventricular failure. J Heart Lung Transplant. 2011;30:1360–7.

133. Belohlavek J., Rohn V., Jansa P., Tosovsky J., Kunstyr J., et al. Veno-arterial ECMO in severe acute right ventricular failure with pulmonary obstructive hemodynamic pattern. J Invasive Cardiol. 2010;22:365–9.

134. Berman M., Tsui S., Vuylsteke A., Klein A., Jenkins DP. Life-threatening right ventricular failure in Pplmonary hypertension: RVAD or ECMO? J Heart Lung Transplant. 2008;27:1188–9.

135. Hamon M., Agostini D., Le Page O., Riddell J., Hamon M. Prognostic impact of right ventricular involvement in patients with acute myocardial infarction: meta-analysis. Crit Care Med 2008; 36: 2023–2033.

136. Keeley E., Boura J. and Grines C. Primary angioplasty versus intravenous thrombolytic therapy for acute myocardial infarction: a quantitative review of 23 randomised trials. Lancet 2003; 361: 13–20.

137. Khan S., Kundi A., Sharieff S. Prevalence of right ventricular myocardial infarction in patients with acute inferior wall myocardial infarction. Int J Clin Pract, 2004 Apr;58(4): 354-7.

138. Miszalski-Jamka T., Klimeczek P., Tomala M., Krupiński M., Zawadowski G., et al., Extent of RV dysfunction and myocardial infarction assessed by CMR are independent outcome predictors early after STEMI treated with primary angioplasty. JACC Cardiovasc Imaging, 2010 Dec;3(12):1237-46.

139. Kukla P., Dudek D., Rakowski T., Dziewierz A., Mielecki W., et al., Inferior wall myocardial infarction with or without right ventricular involvement - treatment and in-hospital course. Kardiol Pol, 2006 64(6):583-8.

140. Gumina R., Murphy J., Rihal C., Lennon R., Wright R. Long-term survival after right ventricular infarction. Am J Cardiol 2006; 98: 1571–1573.

141. Hochman J., Sleeper L., Webb J., Dzavik V., Buller C., et al.; SHOCK Investigators. Early revascularization and long-term survival in cardiogenic shock complicating acute myocardial infarction. JAMA 2006; 295: 2511–2515.

142. Mendes L., Picard M., Sleeper L. Cardiogenic shock: predictors of outcome based on right and left ventricular size and function at presentation. Coron Artery Dis, 2005 Jun;16(4): 209-15.

143. Mehta S., Eikelboom J., Natarajan M., Diaz R., Yi C., et al. Impact of right ventricular involvement on mortality and morbidity in patients with inferior myocardial infarction. J Am Coll Cardiol. 2001;37:37–43.

144. Foussas S., Zairis M., Tsiaousis G., et al., The impact of right ventricular involvement on the postdischarge long-term mortality in patients with acute

inferior ST-segment elevation myocardial infarction. Angiology, 2010 Feb;61(2):179-83.

145. Jim M., Chan A., Tse H., Lau C. Predictors of inhospital outcome after acute inferior wall myocardial infarction. Singapore Med J, 2009 Oct;50(10):956-61.

146. Bodi V., Sanchis J., Mainar L., Chorro FJ., Nunez J., et al., Right ventricular involvement in anterior myocardial infarction: a translational approach. Cardiovascular Research, 2010(87):601-608.

147. Hayrapetyan H. Influence of associated right ventricular infarction on clinical course, prognosis, and ergometric parameters physical tolerance in patients with left ventricular ST segment elevated acute myocardial infarction. The Journal of Heart Disease 2010; 7(1):38.

148. Hayrapetyan H. The effect of right ventricular leisure on the acute phase of left myocardial infarction. Acute Cardiac Care Congress, European Heart Journal 2006; 8(S2):36-37.

149. Hayrapetyan H. Echocardiographic assessement of right ventricle in acute myocardial infarction [Aricle in Russian]. Medical Science of Armenia, 2012. LII(2):58-67.

150. Bueno H., López-Palop R., Pérez-David E., García-García J., López-Sendón J., et al., Combined effect of age and right ventricular involvement on acute inferior myocardial infarction prognosis. Circulation, 1998;98(17):1714-20.

151. Adamyan, K. and H. Hayrapetyan, Influence of involvement of right ventricle in clinical course, prognosis and ergometric parameters in left ventricle inferior ST elevation myocardial infarction [Article in Russian]. Medical Science of Armenia, 2010;4:86-89.

152. Samad B., Alam M., and Jensen-Urstad K. Prognostic impact of right ventricular involvementas assessed by tricuspid annular motion in patients with acute myocardial infarction. Am J Cardiol., 2002. 90(7):778–781.

153. Werf F., Ardissino D., Betriu A., Cokkinos D., Falk E., et al. Management of Acute Myocardial Infarction in patients presenting with ST-segment elevation. European Heart Journal. 2003;24:28-66.

154. Werf F., Bax J., Betriu A., Blomstrom-Lundqvist C., Crea F., et al. Management of acute myocardial infarction in patients presenting with persistent ST-segment elevation. European Heart Journal. 2008;29:2909-2945.

155. O'Gara P., Kushner F., Ascheim D., Casey D., Chung M., et al. 2013 ACCF/AHA Guideline for the Management of ST-Elevation Myocardial Infarction. A Report of the American College of Cardiology

Foundation/American Heart Association Task Force on Practice Guidelines. Circulation. 2013;127:e362-e425.

156. Lang R., Bierig M., Devereux R., Flachskampf F.A., Foster E., et al. Recommendations for chamber quantification: a report from the American Society of Echocardiography's Guidelines and Standards Committee and the Chamber Quantification Writing Group, developed in conjunction with the European Association of Echocardiography, a branch of the European Society of Cardiology. American Society of Echocardiography. 2005;18:1440-1463.

157. Otterstad J. Measuring left ventricular volume and ejection fraction with the biplane Simpson's method. Heart. 2002;88:559-560.

158. Lakoumentas J., Panou F., Kotseroglou V., Aggeli K., Harbis P., et al. The Tei index of myocardial performance: application in cardiology. Hellenic J Cardiol. 2005(46):52-58.

159. Curtis J., Sokol S., Wang Y., Rathore S., Ko D., et al. The association of left ventricular ejection fraction, mortality, and cause of death in stable outpatients with heart failure. J Am Coll Cardiol. 2013;42(4):736-742.

160. Bruch C., Schmermund A., Marin D. Tei index in patients with mild to moderate congestive heart failure. Eur Heart J. 2000(21):1888-1895.

161. Poulsen S., Jensen S., Nielsen J., Møller J., Egstrup K. Serial changes and prognostic implications of a Doppler derived index of combined left ventricular systolic and diastolic myocardial performance in acute myocardial infarction. Am J Cardiol. 2000(85):19-25.

162. Karaye K. Relationship between tei index and left ventricular geometric patterns in a hypertensive population: a cross-sectional study. Cardiovascular Ultrasound. 2011;9(21).

163. Souza L., Campos O., Peres C., Carvalho A. Echocardiographic predictors of early in-hospital heart failure during first ST-elevation acute myocardial infarction: does myocardial performance index and left atrial volume improve diagnosis over conventional parameters of left ventricular function? Cardiovasc Ultrasound. 2011 Jun 3;9(17).

164. Schwammenthal E., Adler Y., Amichai K., Sagie A., Behar S., et al. Prognostic value of global myocardial performance indices in acute myocardial infarction: comparison to measures of systolic and diastolic left ventricular function. Chest. 2003 Nov;124(5):1645-1651.

165. Toufan M., Sajjadieh A-R. Predictive Value of Myocardial Performance Index for Cardiac Events in Patients Hospitalized for First Myocardial Infarction. Research Journal of Biological Sciences. 2008;3(6):589-595.

166. Vizzardi E., D'Aloia A., Bordonali T., Bugatti S., Piovanelli B., al. Long-Term Prognostic Value of the Right Ventricular Myocardial Performance Index Compared to Other Indexes of Right Ventricular Function in Patients with Moderate Chronic Heart Failure. Echocardiography. 2012;29(7):773-778.

167. Engström A., Vis M., Bouma B., van den Brink R., Baan J Jr., et al. Right ventricular dysfunction is an independent predictor for mortality in ST-elevation myocardial infarction patients presenting with cardiogenic shock on admission. Eur J Heart Fail. 2010 Mar;12(3):276-282.

168. Antoni M., Scherptong R., Atary J., Atary J., Boersmaet E., et al. Prognostic value of right ventricular function in patients after acute myocardial infarction treated with primary percutaneous coronary intervention. Circ Cardiovasc Imaging. 2010 May;3(3):264-271

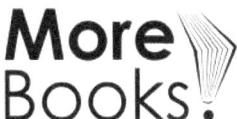
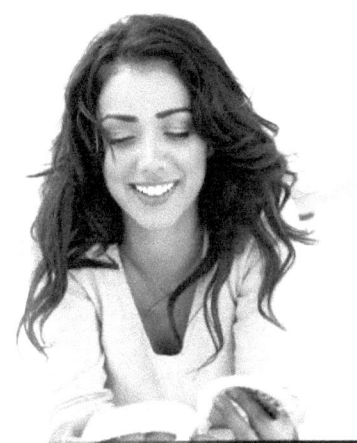
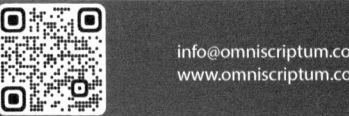
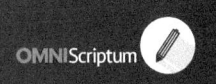

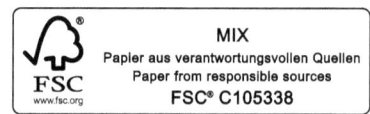
Printed by Books on Demand GmbH, Norderstedt / Germany